OWEN HUNTER

The Healthy Aging Handbook

Contents

INTRODUCTION

As we grow older, the prospect of aging can evoke a range of emotions – from excitement about new experiences and opportunities to apprehension about the challenges that may lie ahead. However, the narrative surrounding aging is rapidly shifting. Rather than viewing it as a time of inevitable decline, we now understand that healthy aging is not only achievable but can be an incredibly rewarding and empowering phase of life.

In today's world, life expectancy continues to rise, and many of us can look forward to spending more time in our golden years than previous generations. This presents a remarkable opportunity to redefine the aging experience and to embrace the remarkable potential that comes with growing older. The Healthy Aging Handbook is your comprehensive guide to navigating this new frontier, equipping you with the knowledge, tools, and strategies to thrive as you age.

Debunking the Myths of Aging

For far too long, aging has been shrouded in misconceptions and negative stereotypes. The common perception of older adults as frail, sedentary, and mentally declining is simply not reflective of the vibrant, active, and intellectually engaged individuals we see all around us. It's time to shatter these outdated myths and embrace a more positive and empowering perspective on the aging process.

One of the most pervasive myths is that physical and cognitive decline are an inevitable consequence of growing older. While it's true that certain changes do occur as we age, the rate and degree of these changes are heavily influenced by our lifestyle choices and overall health. Through proper nutrition, regular exercise, and brain-stimulating activities, we can maintain our physical and mental capacities well into our later years.

Another myth is that older adults are resistant to change and unable to adapt to new technologies or ways of life. In reality, many older adults are embracing lifelong learning, exploring new hobbies and skills, and readily adapting to the digital age. With the right mindset and support, older adults can continue to grow, evolve, and contribute to their communities in meaningful ways.

It's also commonly believed that retirement is the end of a productive and fulfilling life. On the contrary, retirement can be an exciting transition that opens up new opportunities for personal growth, volunteerism, and encore careers. By reframing retirement as a chance to pursue passions and reinvent ourselves, we can find immense satisfaction and purpose in this next chapter of our lives.

The Benefits of Healthy Aging

When we reject the negative stereotypes and embrace the true potential of aging, we unlock a world of remarkable benefits. Healthy aging is not just about maintaining physical and cognitive function – it's about thriving in all aspects of life, from emotional well-being to financial security and social engagement.

Perhaps one of the most significant benefits of healthy aging is the preservation of independence and autonomy. By taking proactive steps to maintain our health and vitality, we can minimize the risk of debilitating conditions and remain self-sufficient for longer. This allows us to continue living in our own homes, pursuing our hobbies, and making our own decisions – all of which are essential for maintaining a high quality of life.

Healthy aging also supports emotional well-being and psychological resilience. As we grow older, we have the opportunity to cultivate rich, meaningful relationships, develop a deeper understanding of ourselves, and find greater purpose and fulfillment in our lives. By managing stress, practicing mindfulness, and engaging in activities that nurture our emotional and social needs, we can experience a profound sense of inner peace and contentment.

Furthermore, healthy aging can have a positive impact on our financial security and long-term wellbeing. By adopting healthy habits and proactively managing our health, we can reduce the risk of costly medical expenses and safeguard our financial resources for retirement. This, in turn, allows us to enjoy a greater sense of financial independence and the freedom to pursue our passions and dreams.

Perhaps most importantly, healthy aging empowers us to leave a lasting legacy and inspire others. As we grow older, we have the opportunity to share our wisdom, mentor younger generations, and contribute to our communities in meaningful ways. By embracing healthy aging and setting a positive example, we can inspire others to follow in our footsteps and create a ripple effect of wellbeing that benefits us all.

Your Guide to Thriving in the Golden Years

The Healthy Aging Handbook is your comprehensive roadmap to navigating the exciting and rewarding journey of growing older. Whether you are in your 50s, 60s, 70s, or beyond, this book will provide you with the knowledge, tools, and strategies to optimize your physical, mental, emotional, and social well-being.

Throughout the chapters that follow, you will discover a wealth of information and practical guidance on a wide range of topics essential for healthy aging, including:

- Nutrition and dietary recommendations for older adults
- The role of physical activity and exercise in maintaining mobility and vitality
- Strategies for preserving cognitive function and brain health
- Techniques for managing stress, anxiety, and emotional well-being
- The importance of quality sleep and how to improve sleep habits
- Proactive healthcare measures and preventive screenings
- The integration of holistic approaches and supplements
- Creating age-friendly environments and accessing community resources
- Financial planning and retirement strategies
- Caregiving support and building a strong support network
- Embracing lifelong learning and personal growth opportunities
- Celebrating the positive aspects of aging and leaving a lasting legacy

By exploring these essential topics, you will gain a comprehensive understanding of the multifaceted nature of healthy aging. More importantly, you will be empowered to take proactive steps to enhance your overall well-being and thrive in the years to come.

A New Era of Healthy Aging

We are living in a remarkable era of longevity, where the prospect of enjoying a longer, healthier, and more fulfilling life is within our reach. However, this new era of healthy aging requires a fundamental shift in our mindset and approach to growing older.

Rather than passively accepting the conventional narratives of aging, we must actively embrace the power of personal responsibility and lifestyle choices. By making informed decisions about our health, our finances, our social connections, and our personal growth, we can shape the trajectory of our own aging experience.

The Healthy Aging Handbook is your invitation to embark on this transformative journey. Within these pages, you will discover the keys to unlocking your full potential and living your best life, no matter your age. Whether you are already well on your path to healthy aging or just beginning to explore the possibilities, this book will equip you with the knowledge and inspiration to navigate the exciting years ahead.

As you read on, keep an open mind and a willingness to challenge the status quo. Embrace the notion that aging is not a passive experience, but rather a dynamic and empowering process in which you are the driving force. With the right mindset, the right tools, and the right support, you can not only meet the challenges of aging but transcend them, emerging as a vibrant, engaged, and fulfilled individual.

The future of aging is ours to define. Let's rewrite the narrative together and create a world where healthy aging is the norm, not the exception. Join us on this transformative journey, and discover the boundless possibilities that await you in the golden years.

CHAPTER 1

Chapter 1: The Importance of Healthy Aging

As we embark on this journey of healthy aging, it's essential to first understand the profound significance and far-reaching benefits of this pursuit. Healthy aging is not merely about maintaining physical health or delaying the onset of age-related diseases – it's about thriving in all aspects of life, from mental and emotional well-being to social engagement and financial security.

In this opening chapter, we will explore the compelling reasons why healthy aging should be a top priority for individuals of all ages. We will delve into the personal, societal, and global implications of embracing a proactive approach to growing older, and how the choices we make today can profoundly shape the quality of our lives in the years to come.

The Personal Rewards of Healthy Aging

At its core, healthy aging is about reclaiming control over our own destinies and ensuring that we have the physical, mental, and emotional resources to live life to the fullest. By making a concerted effort to prioritize our well-being, we can unlock a world of personal rewards and enriching experiences.

Preserving Independence and Autonomy

One of the most significant benefits of healthy aging is the preservation of independence and autonomy. As we grow older, the ability to perform everyday tasks, make our own decisions, and maintain an active lifestyle becomes increasingly important for our overall quality of life. By taking proactive steps to maintain our physical and cognitive function, we can minimize the risk of debilitating conditions and remain self-sufficient for longer.

This not only allows us to continue living in our own homes and communities but also empowers us to pursue our passions, engage in hobbies, and participate in the activities that bring us joy and fulfillment. When we are able to maintain our independence, we retain a greater sense of control over our lives and the freedom to make choices that align with our personal values and preferences.

Enhancing Emotional Well-being and Resilience

Healthy aging is not just about physical health – it's also about nurturing our emotional and psychological well-being. As we grow older, we have the opportunity to cultivate a deeper understanding of ourselves, develop more meaningful relationships, and find greater purpose and fulfillment in our lives.

By adopting strategies to manage stress, cultivate positive emotions, and engage in activities that nourish our emotional needs, we can experience a profound sense of inner peace, contentment, and resilience. This, in turn, can help us better navigate the challenges and transitions that often come with aging, allowing us to approach the golden years with a greater sense of emotional stability and adaptability.

Maintaining Cognitive Sharpness and Mental Acuity

One of the most common concerns about aging is the potential for cognitive decline and memory loss. While some changes in brain function are natural as we grow older, research has shown that we can take proactive steps to maintain and even enhance our cognitive abilities through engaging in mentally stimulating activities, learning new skills, and adopting healthy lifestyle habits.

By prioritizing brain health and engaging in regular brain-boosting exercises, we can preserve our mental sharpness, problem-solving skills, and decision-making capacities well into our later years. This not only allows us to continue enjoying intellectually stimulating pursuits but also helps us remain independent, adaptive, and engaged with the world around us.

Improving Physical Health and Wellness

Perhaps the most obvious benefit of healthy aging is the preservation of physical health and wellness. By incorporating regular exercise, proper nutrition, and preventive healthcare into our daily lives, we can reduce the risk of age-related diseases, maintain our mobility and flexibility, and enjoy a greater sense of physical vitality.

When we take care of our bodies, we are not only improving our immediate well-being but also investing in our long-term quality of life. By minimizing the impact of chronic conditions and reducing the need for medical interventions, we can enjoy more active, fulfilling, and independent years as we grow older.

Enhancing Financial Security and Stability

Healthy aging also has significant implications for our financial well-being and long-term security. By proactively managing our health and reducing the risk of costly medical expenses, we can safeguard our financial resources and enjoy greater peace of mind in retirement.

Moreover, the personal rewards of healthy aging – such as maintaining independence, emotional resilience, and cognitive function – can translate into increased earning potential, the ability to continue working or pursue encore careers, and the opportunity to make the most of our retirement years without the burden of debilitating health concerns.

The Societal Benefits of Healthy Aging

The advantages of healthy aging extend far beyond the individual – they also have profound implications for the larger social fabric. As the population of older adults continues to grow, the collective impact of healthy aging can reshape communities, strengthen social support systems, and contribute to a more prosperous and equitable society.

Reducing the Burden on Healthcare Systems

One of the most significant societal benefits of healthy aging is the potential to alleviate the strain on healthcare systems. By maintaining our health and reducing the incidence of age-related diseases, we can minimize the demand for costly medical interventions, hospitalizations, and long-term care.

This, in turn, allows healthcare resources to be more efficiently allocated, enabling healthcare providers to focus on delivering high-quality, personalized care to those who need it the most. Furthermore, a healthier aging population can lead to lower healthcare costs for individuals, families, and the broader community, making the healthcare system more sustainable and accessible for all.

Fostering Intergenerational Connections and Understanding

Embracing healthy aging can also play a crucial role in strengthening the bonds between generations and promoting greater understanding and respect. As older adults maintain their physical, mental, and social vitality, they are better equipped to actively participate in their communities, share their wisdom and experiences, and serve as mentors and role models for younger generations.

This intergenerational exchange can foster a deeper appreciation for the diverse perspectives and life experiences that each age group brings to the table. It can also inspire younger individuals to adopt healthier lifestyles and consider the long-term implications of their choices, ultimately creating a ripple effect of well-being that benefits people of all ages.

Enhancing Workforce Participation and Economic Productivity

Healthy aging can also have a positive impact on workforce participation and economic productivity. As older adults maintain their cognitive abilities, physical stamina, and adaptability, they can continue to make valuable contributions to the workforce, either in their current roles or through encore careers and entrepreneurial ventures.

This not only taps into the wealth of knowledge and experience that older adults possess but also helps to address labor shortages and skill gaps that many industries are facing. By encouraging and supporting the continued participation of older adults in the workforce, we can foster a more diverse, experienced, and productive economic landscape that benefits both individuals and the broader community.

Promoting Inclusive and Age-Friendly Communities

Healthy aging is not just about individual well-being – it's also about creating communities that are inclusive, accessible, and supportive of people of all ages. By designing public spaces, transportation systems, and housing options that cater to the needs of older adults, we can ensure that everyone has the opportunity to participate fully in community life, access essential services, and maintain their independence.

Moreover, age-friendly communities that prioritize the well-being of older adults can have a positive ripple effect, improving the quality of life for people of all ages. This can lead to a more vibrant, interconnected, and equitable society where individuals of all generations can thrive and contribute to the common good.

The Global Significance of Healthy Aging

The importance of healthy aging extends beyond the individual and societal levels – it has far-reaching implications for the global community as well. As the world's population continues to age, the collective impact of healthy aging can shape the future of healthcare, social support systems, and sustainable development on an international scale.

Addressing the Challenge of an Aging Global Population

One of the most significant global trends of the 21st century is the rapid aging of the world's population. According to the World Health Organization, the number of people aged 60 years and older is expected to more than double, from 1 billion in 2020 to 2.1 billion by 2050. This demographic shift presents both challenges and opportunities for the global community.

By embracing healthy aging on a global scale, we can help mitigate the strain on healthcare systems, social support networks, and economic infrastructures that this aging population could otherwise create. By empowering older adults to maintain their health, independence, and active participation in society, we can ensure that the benefits of longevity are realized by individuals, communities, and nations around the world.

Promoting Sustainable Development and Inclusive Growth

The principles of healthy aging are closely aligned with the United Nations' Sustainable Development Goals (SDGs), which aim to create a more equitable, prosperous, and environmentally sustainable future for all. By investing in the well-being of older adults, we can contribute to the achievement of several key SDGs, including good health and well-being, reduced inequalities, and sustainable cities and communities.

Moreover, by fostering healthy aging on a global scale, we can help to create more inclusive and age-friendly societies that provide equal opportunities for people of all ages to participate in economic, social, and civic life. This, in turn, can lead to more sustainable and equitable development that benefits individuals, families, and communities around the world.

Enhancing Global Health and Resilience

Healthy aging also has important implications for global health and resilience. By promoting preventive healthcare, physical activity, and healthy lifestyle habits, we can help reduce the incidence of non-communicable diseases, such as cardiovascular disease, diabetes, and certain types of cancer, which disproportionately affect older populations.

Furthermore, individuals who have adopted healthy aging practices are often better equipped to withstand and recover from external shocks, such as natural disasters, pandemics, and economic downturns. By cultivating physical, mental, and emotional resilience, we can contribute to the overall health and well-being of the global community, ultimately enhancing our collective ability to navigate and overcome the challenges of the future.

Embracing the Power of Healthy Aging

As we have explored in this chapter, the importance of healthy aging cannot be overstated. From the personal rewards of maintaining independence and well-being to the broader societal and global implications, the choices we make today can have a profound and lasting impact on our lives and the lives of those around us.

By recognizing the significance of healthy aging and making it a top priority, we can unlock a world of possibilities and create a future where growing older is celebrated, not feared. Whether you are just beginning to explore the concept of healthy aging or have already taken steps to enhance your well-being, this handbook will provide you with the knowledge, tools, and inspiration to thrive in the golden years and beyond.

In the chapters that follow, we will delve deeper into the various facets of healthy aging, equipping you with the strategies and resources to optimize your physical, mental, emotional, and social well-being. Through a comprehensive, evidence-based approach, we will empower you to take control of your own aging experience and create a fulfilling, rewarding, and impactful life in the years to come.

Remember, the future of aging is ours to define. By embracing healthy aging and sharing our experiences with others, we can inspire a global movement that transforms the way we think about growing older. So, let's embark on this journey together, and unlock the boundless potential that awaits us in the golden years.

CHAPTER 2

Chapter 2: Nutrition for Healthy Aging

As we journey through the golden years, our nutritional needs and dietary habits play a critical role in maintaining our overall health and well-being. While the principles of healthy eating remain important throughout our lives, the specific nutritional requirements and considerations for older adults can vary significantly from those of younger individuals.

In this chapter, we will explore the foundational pillars of nutrition for healthy aging, examining the unique macronutrient and micronutrient needs of older adults, as well as the dietary strategies that can help support physical vitality, cognitive function, and disease prevention. By understanding the science behind healthy aging nutrition, you will be empowered to make informed choices that nourish your body, mind, and spirit, setting the stage for a fulfilling and vibrant future.

Macronutrients for Older Adults

Macronutrients – the three primary types of nutrients that provide the body with energy (calories) – are essential for maintaining optimal health as we age. However, the specific ratios and quantities of these macronutrients may need to be adjusted to address the unique physiological changes and requirements of older adults.

Protein: Preserving Muscle Mass and Function

Protein is a vital macronutrient for older adults, as it plays a crucial role in maintaining and building muscle mass, supporting bone health, and preserving overall physical function. As we age, we naturally experience a gradual decline in muscle mass and strength, a condition known as sarcopenia. This can lead to reduced mobility, increased risk of falls, and a diminished ability to perform everyday tasks.

To combat this age-related muscle loss, the recommended dietary protein intake for older adults is generally higher than the recommendations for younger individuals. The current guidelines suggest that older adults should consume between 1.2 and 1.5 grams of protein per kilogram of body weight per day, depending on their level of physical activity and overall health status.

Incorporating a variety of high-quality protein sources, such as lean meats, poultry, fish, eggs, dairy products, legumes, and nuts, can help older adults meet their protein needs and support the maintenance of muscle mass and function. Additionally, the strategic timing of protein intake, such as consuming protein-rich meals or supplements before and after exercise, can further enhance the muscle-building and preserving effects.

Carbohydrates: Fuel for Energy and Brain Function

Carbohydrates are the body's primary source of energy, and they play a vital role in supporting cognitive function, maintaining blood sugar levels, and providing the fuel needed for physical activity. For older adults, the recommended intake of carbohydrates is generally similar to that of younger adults, with the emphasis shifting towards complex, fiber-rich carbohydrates.

Complex carbohydrates, such as those found in whole grains, fruits, vegetables, and legumes, are more slowly digested and absorbed, helping to regulate blood sugar levels and promote a steady supply of energy throughout the day.

These carbohydrate sources are also rich in essential vitamins, minerals, and antioxidants that can support overall health and well-being.

In contrast, simple or refined carbohydrates, such as those found in added sugars, white bread, and processed snacks, can contribute to blood sugar spikes and crashes, potentially leading to fatigue, mood swings, and an increased risk of chronic diseases like type 2 diabetes. By focusing on nutrient-dense, complex carbohydrate sources, older adults can maintain stable energy levels, support brain function, and promote overall metabolic health.

Healthy Fats: Supporting Brain, Heart, and Joint Health

Fats are another essential macronutrient for older adults, playing a crucial role in maintaining brain health, supporting cardiovascular function, and reducing inflammation in the body. Unlike the common misconception that all fats are harmful, certain types of healthy fats can provide numerous benefits as we age.

Unsaturated fats, such as those found in avocados, nuts, seeds, and fatty fish, are particularly important for older adults. These fats can help lower the risk of heart disease, improve cognitive function, and reduce joint pain and inflammation associated with conditions like osteoarthritis.

In contrast, saturated and trans fats, which are often found in processed foods, baked goods, and fried items, can contribute to an increased risk of heart disease, stroke, and other chronic health issues. By emphasizing healthy, unsaturated fats in the diet and limiting the intake of saturated and trans fats, older adults can support cardiovascular, brain, and joint health.

Micronutrients and Antioxidants for Healthy Aging

In addition to macronutrients, the proper intake of micronutrients and antioxidants is crucial for maintaining optimal health and well-being as we age. These essential vitamins, minerals, and plant-based compounds play a vital role in supporting immune function, cognitive performance, bone health, and the body's natural defense against oxidative stress and inflammation.

Vitamins and Minerals

As we grow older, our bodies may become less efficient at absorbing and utilizing certain vitamins and minerals, making it essential to ensure adequate intake through our diets or targeted supplementation.

Some key micronutrients that deserve special attention for older adults include:

- Vitamin D: This essential vitamin is crucial for maintaining bone health and supporting immune function. Many older adults may have insufficient vitamin D levels due to decreased sun exposure and reduced ability to synthesize vitamin D in the skin.
  - Vitamin B12: Responsible for red blood cell formation, nerve function, and energy production, vitamin B12 deficiency is common in older adults, particularly those taking certain medications or with digestive issues.
  - Calcium: A vital mineral for bone health, calcium is essential for preventing osteoporosis and reducing the risk of falls and fractures in older adults.
  - Magnesium: This mineral plays a key role in muscle and nerve function, blood sugar regulation, and bone health, and may be lacking in the diets of some older individuals.
  - Zinc: Crucial for immune function, wound healing, and taste and smell perception, zinc deficiency can be a concern for older adults, especially those with decreased appetite or underlying health conditions.

By focusing on nutrient-dense, whole-food sources of these and other essential vitamins and minerals, or considering targeted supplementation under the guidance of a healthcare professional, older adults can help ensure they are meeting their micronutrient needs for optimal health and well-being.

Antioxidants and Phytonutrients

In addition to vitamins and minerals, antioxidants and phytonutrients found in plant-based foods can provide significant benefits for healthy aging. These compounds help neutralize the harmful effects of free radicals and oxidative stress, which can contribute to the development of chronic diseases, cognitive decline, and accelerated aging.

Some of the most important antioxidants and phytonutrients for older adults include:

- Carotenoids: Found in brightly colored fruits and vegetables, such as carrots, sweet potatoes, and leafy greens, carotenoids like lutein and zeaxanthin can support eye health and cognitive function.
- Polyphenols: These powerful plant compounds, found in berries, green tea, dark chocolate, and many other plant-based foods, can help reduce inflammation, improve cardiovascular health, and support brain function.
- Resveratrol: This antioxidant, found in the skin of grapes and red wine, has been studied for its potential to support longevity, reduce the risk of chronic diseases, and promote healthy aging.
- Curcumin: The active compound in turmeric, curcumin has been shown to possess anti-inflammatory and neuroprotective properties that may benefit older adults.

By incorporating a variety of colorful, plant-based foods into their diets, older adults can ensure they are obtaining a rich array of beneficial antioxidants and phytonutrients to support their overall health and well-being.

Dietary Recommendations for Healthy Aging

With an understanding of the unique macronutrient and micronutrient needs of older adults, we can now explore the dietary recommendations and strategies that can help support healthy aging. By focusing on a nutrient-dense, balanced approach to eating, older adults can optimize their physical, cognitive, and emotional well-being.

Emphasize Whole, Unprocessed Foods

One of the fundamental principles of healthy aging nutrition is to prioritize whole, minimally processed foods as the foundation of the diet. These nutrient-dense foods, such as fruits, vegetables, whole grains, lean proteins, and healthy fats, provide a rich array of essential vitamins, minerals, fiber, and antioxidants that can support overall health and well-being.

In contrast, highly processed, packaged foods that are high in added sugars, unhealthy fats, and artificial additives can contribute to a range of health issues, including obesity, chronic inflammation, and an increased risk of chronic diseases. By minimizing the intake of these processed foods and focusing on whole, unprocessed options, older adults can nourish their bodies and support healthy aging.

Ensure Adequate Protein Intake

As discussed earlier, protein is a crucial macronutrient for older adults, as it plays a vital role in maintaining muscle mass, supporting bone health, and preserving physical function. To meet their higher protein needs, older adults should aim to consume a variety of high-quality protein sources at each meal, such as lean meats, poultry, fish, eggs, dairy products, legumes, and nuts.

In addition to incorporating protein-rich foods, older adults may also benefit from the strategic use of protein supplements, such as whey, casein, or plant-based proteins, particularly in the context of resistance training or to support muscle recovery and growth. Consulting with a healthcare professional or registered dietitian can help determine the appropriate protein intake and supplementation strategy for an individual's specific needs and goals.

Focus on Fiber-Rich Carbohydrates

As mentioned earlier, complex, fiber-rich carbohydrates should be the primary source of carbohydrates in the diets of older adults. These nutrient-dense options, such as whole grains, fruits, vegetables, and legumes, provide a steady supply of energy, promote healthy blood sugar regulation, and support digestive and cardiovascular health.

Older adults should aim to consume a variety of these fiber-rich carbohydrate sources throughout the day, while limiting the intake of refined or added sugars, which can contribute to blood sugar spikes, energy crashes, and an increased risk of chronic diseases. By emphasizing complex carbohydrates, older adults can maintain stable energy levels, support cognitive function, and promote overall metabolic health.

Incorporate Healthy Fats

Healthy fats, such as those found in avocados, nuts, seeds, and fatty fish, should be a regular part of the older adult's diet. These unsaturated fats can help support brain health, reduce inflammation, and lower the risk of cardiovascular disease.

In addition to incorporating healthy fats into meals and snacks, older adults should be mindful of limiting their intake of saturated and trans fats, which are often found in processed foods, baked goods, and fried items. By focusing on nutrient-dense, unsaturated fat sources, older adults can optimize their heart health, cognitive function, and overall well-being.

Hydrate Adequately

Proper hydration is essential for older adults, as the body's ability to regulate fluid balance can diminish with age. Dehydration can lead to a range of health issues, including fatigue, confusion, constipation, and an increased risk of falls.

Older adults should aim to drink plenty of water and other hydrating fluids throughout the day, such as herbal tea, low-fat milk, or watery fruits and vegetables. The recommended daily fluid intake for older adults is generally around 11.5 cups (2.7 liters) for women and 15.5 cups (3.7 liters) for men, but individual needs may vary based on factors such as climate, physical activity, and health status.

Consider Nutritional Supplements

While a well-balanced, nutrient-dense diet should be the foundation of healthy aging nutrition, older adults may also benefit from the strategic use of targeted nutritional supplements. This can be particularly important for individuals with specific dietary restrictions, underlying health conditions, or increased nutrient needs due to factors such as medication use or malabsorption.

Some common nutritional supplements that may be beneficial for older adults include:

- Vitamin D: To support bone health and immune function
  - Vitamin B12: To address potential deficiencies and support red blood cell formation and nerve function
  - Calcium: To maintain bone density and reduce the risk of osteoporosis
  - Omega-3 fatty acids: To support heart and brain health
  - Probiotic supplements: To promote gut health and immune function

It is essential for older adults to consult with a healthcare professional or registered dietitian before starting any new supplement regimen, as they can help determine the appropriate type, dosage, and timing of supplements based on individual needs and health status.

Embracing a Holistic Approach to Nutrition for Healthy Aging

Healthy aging nutrition is not just about the specific nutrients we consume – it's about adopting a holistic, balanced approach to eating that nourishes our bodies, minds, and spirits. By incorporating mindful eating practices, enjoying the social and cultural aspects of food, and finding joy in the culinary experience, older adults can enhance their overall well-being and create a positive, sustainable relationship with food.

Some key elements of this holistic approach to healthy aging nutrition include:

- Mindful eating: Taking the time to savor and appreciate each meal, being present with the food, and listening to internal hunger and fullness cues.
- Shared mealtimes: Engaging in regular, enjoyable meals with family, friends, or a community, which can foster social connections and emotional fulfillment.
- Culturally meaningful foods: Incorporating traditional, culturally relevant dishes and flavors that connect us to our heritage and provide a sense of belonging.
- Cooking and food preparation: Engaging in the process of preparing meals, which can stimulate cognitive function, fine motor skills, and a sense of accomplishment.
- Flexibility and moderation: Allowing for occasional indulgences and enjoying a variety of foods in moderation, rather than adhering to strict, restrictive diets.

By embracing this holistic approach to nutrition, older adults can create a sustainable, enjoyable, and beneficial relationship with food that supports their overall health and well-being throughout the golden years and beyond.

CHAPTER 3

Chapter 3: Physical Activity and Exercise

As we navigate the journey of healthy aging, regular physical activity and exercise play a crucial role in maintaining our physical, mental, and emotional well-being. While the benefits of an active lifestyle are important at any age, they become increasingly vital as we grow older, helping us to preserve our independence, prevent chronic diseases, and enhance our overall quality of life.

In this chapter, we will delve into the pivotal role of physical activity and exercise in the context of healthy aging. We will explore the various components of an effective exercise regimen, including strength training, cardiovascular fitness, and flexibility, and discuss practical strategies for adapting and incorporating these activities into your daily routine. By the end of this chapter, you will be equipped with the knowledge and inspiration to embark on a fulfilling and transformative journey of physical and mental rejuvenation.

The Importance of Physical Activity and Exercise for Older Adults

As we age, our bodies naturally undergo a range of physiological changes, including a gradual decline in muscle mass, bone density, and cardiovascular function. Without regular physical activity, these age-related changes can accelerate, leading to a loss of mobility, increased risk of falls and injuries, and a higher susceptibility to chronic health conditions.

However, by embracing an active lifestyle and incorporating a well-rounded exercise regimen into our daily lives, we can counteract many of these age-related declines and maintain our physical, mental, and emotional well-being well into our golden years.

Preserving Muscular Strength and Mobility

One of the primary benefits of regular physical activity for older adults is the preservation of muscular strength and mobility. As we mentioned in the previous chapter, the gradual loss of muscle mass and strength, known as sarcopenia, is a common consequence of aging. This can lead to reduced mobility, increased risk of falls, and a diminished ability to perform everyday tasks.

By engaging in strength training exercises, such as resistance training with weights or resistance bands, older adults can combat the effects of sarcopenia and maintain their muscle mass, strength, and overall physical function. This, in turn, can help them to remain independent, active, and able to participate in the activities they enjoy, enhancing their overall quality of life.

Improving Cardiovascular Health and Endurance

In addition to maintaining muscular strength, regular physical activity also plays a crucial role in supporting cardiovascular health and endurance. As we age, our cardiovascular system can become less efficient, leading to an increased risk of heart disease, stroke, and other related conditions.

By incorporating cardiovascular exercises, such as brisk walking, swimming, or cycling, into their fitness regimen, older adults can improve their heart health, lower their blood pressure, and enhance their overall endurance and stamina. This can not only reduce the risk of cardiovascular events but also enable them to engage in more physically demanding activities and maintain their independence for longer.

Enhancing Cognitive Function and Emotional Well-being

Physical activity and exercise are not only beneficial for our physical health but also have a profound impact on our cognitive function and emotional well-being. Regular physical activity has been shown to improve mood, reduce the risk of depression and anxiety, and support cognitive abilities, such as memory, problem-solving, and decision-making.

This is particularly important for older adults, as they may be more susceptible to cognitive decline and mental health challenges due to factors such as social isolation, chronic stress, and age-related changes in the brain. By engaging in physical activity, older adults can stimulate the release of feel-good neurotransmitters, improve blood flow to the brain, and support the growth and development of new neural connections, all of which can contribute to enhanced cognitive function and emotional well-being.

Reducing the Risk of Chronic Diseases

Perhaps one of the most significant benefits of regular physical activity for older adults is its ability to reduce the risk of chronic diseases. Conditions such as type 2 diabetes, certain types of cancer, and Alzheimer's disease have all been shown to be positively impacted by an active lifestyle.

By engaging in a variety of physical activities, older adults can improve their metabolic function, strengthen their immune system, and reduce the inflammatory processes that can contribute to the development of chronic diseases. This, in turn, can help them maintain their health, independence, and quality of life for longer, reducing the burden on healthcare systems and allowing them to fully enjoy their golden years.

Components of an Effective Exercise Regimen for Older Adults

To reap the full benefits of physical activity and exercise, it's essential for older adults to incorporate a well-rounded and balanced exercise regimen into their daily lives. This should include a combination of strength training, cardiovascular fitness, and flexibility exercises, each of which plays a crucial role in supporting overall health and well-being.

Strength Training: Maintaining Muscle Mass and Bone Health

As we discussed earlier, strength training is a critical component of healthy aging, as it helps to maintain and even build muscle mass, which in turn supports physical function, mobility, and independence. Older adults should aim to incorporate strength training exercises, such as resistance training with weights, resistance bands, or bodyweight exercises, into their routine at least two to three times per week.

These strength-building activities can target all the major muscle groups, including the arms, legs, core, and back, and can be tailored to individual fitness levels and abilities. For older adults, it's particularly important to focus on exercises that challenge the major muscle groups, as these movements can have a more significant impact on overall strength and physical function.

In addition to maintaining muscle mass, strength training can also help to preserve bone density, which is crucial for reducing the risk of osteoporosis and preventing falls and fractures. By incorporating weight-bearing exercises into their routine, older adults can stimulate the growth and maintenance of strong, healthy bones, further enhancing their physical resilience and independence.

Cardiovascular Fitness: Improving Heart Health and Endurance

Cardiovascular exercises, such as brisk walking, swimming, cycling, or dancing, are essential for maintaining a healthy heart, lungs, and circulatory system. Older adults should aim to engage in moderate-intensity cardiovascular activities for at least 150 minutes per week, or more vigorous activities for at least 75 minutes per week.

These cardiovascular exercises not only improve heart health and reduce the risk of cardiovascular diseases but also enhance overall endurance, enabling older adults to maintain an active lifestyle and participate in a wider range of physical activities. Additionally, many cardiovascular exercises can be enjoyed with friends or in a group setting, providing both physical and social benefits.

It's important to note that older adults should consult with their healthcare provider before starting or significantly increasing their cardiovascular exercise regimen, as they may need to consider any underlying health conditions or medication interactions that could affect their exercise tolerance or safety.

Flexibility and Balance: Improving Mobility and Reducing Fall Risk

In addition to strength training and cardiovascular exercises, older adults should also incorporate flexibility and balance exercises into their fitness routine. These activities, such as stretching, yoga, tai chi, or Pilates, can help to maintain and improve range of motion, joint flexibility, and balance, all of which are crucial for reducing the risk of falls and injuries.

As we age, our flexibility and balance can naturally decline, leading to increased stiffness, reduced mobility, and a higher risk of falls and fractures. By engaging in regular flexibility and balance exercises, older adults can improve their stability, coordination, and range of motion, allowing them to move more freely and safely throughout their daily activities.

Many flexibility and balance exercises can also have a calming, meditative effect, which can benefit both physical and mental well-being. Older adults may find these types of activities particularly enjoyable and accessible, as they can often be performed at a slower pace and with a focus on mindfulness and relaxation.

Strategies for Incorporating Physical Activity into Daily Life

While the benefits of physical activity and exercise for older adults are well-established, the actual implementation of an effective fitness routine can sometimes be a challenge. Factors such as limited mobility, chronic health conditions, or a lack of motivation can all pose barriers to regular physical activity.

However, with a little creativity and a willingness to adapt, older adults can find ways to incorporate physical activity into their daily lives in a sustainable and enjoyable manner. Here are some strategies to consider:

Start Slowly and Build Up Gradually

For older adults who are new to regular exercise or have been inactive for some time, it's essential to start slowly and build up their physical activity levels gradually. This can help to prevent injury, minimize soreness, and foster a positive and sustainable exercise habit.

Begin with simple, low-impact activities, such as gentle stretching, light walking, or chair-based exercises, and gradually increase the duration, intensity, and variety of your workouts over time. This incremental approach can help to build confidence, improve fitness, and reduce the risk of discouragement or burnout.

Find Activities You Enjoy

One of the keys to maintaining a consistent exercise routine is to find physical activities that you genuinely enjoy. This could be anything from swimming, dancing, or gardening to joining a local hiking group or participating in a community exercise class.

By focusing on activities that you find fun, engaging, and meaningful, you're more likely to stick with your exercise regimen and reap the full benefits of an active lifestyle. Additionally, engaging in social or group-based activities can provide an extra layer of motivation and support, further enhancing the enjoyment and sustainability of your fitness journey.

Incorporate Physical Activity into Your Daily Routine

Another effective strategy for older adults is to find ways to integrate physical activity into their daily routines, rather than treating it as a separate or standalone task. This can involve simple adjustments, such as taking the stairs instead of the elevator, going for a brisk walk during your lunch break, or doing stretches or light exercises while watching television.

By weaving physical activity into your everyday life, you can make exercise a natural and seamless part of your day, reducing the perceived burden or effort required to maintain an active lifestyle. This approach can be particularly beneficial for older adults who may have limited time or mobility, as it allows them to accumulate physical activity throughout the day without feeling overwhelmed.

Adapt and Modify Exercises as Needed

As we age, our physical capabilities and limitations may change, and it's important to be flexible and adaptable in our approach to exercise. If certain activities become too challenging or cause discomfort, don't hesitate to modify or substitute them with alternative exercises that better suit your current abilities and needs.

This may involve using assistive equipment, such as resistance bands or stability balls, or finding low-impact variations of exercises. It's also crucial to listen to your body and be willing to adjust the duration, intensity, or frequency of your workouts as necessary to prevent injury and ensure a safe and enjoyable exercise experience.

Enlist the Support of Others

Embarking on a fitness journey can be more enjoyable and sustainable when you have the support and encouragement of others. Consider inviting family members, friends, or neighbors to join you in your physical activity routines, or seek out local exercise classes or community groups that cater to older adults.

Alternatively, you can enlist the help of a personal trainer or physical therapist who specializes in working with older adults. These professionals can provide personalized guidance, motivation, and accountability to help you achieve your fitness goals safely and effectively.

Overcoming Common Barriers to Physical Activity

While the benefits of physical activity for older adults are clear, there are often challenges and barriers that can make it difficult to maintain a consistent exercise routine. Understanding and addressing these barriers can be crucial for developing a sustainable, long-term approach to healthy aging through physical fitness.

Limited Mobility or Chronic Health Conditions

For older adults with limited mobility or chronic health conditions, such as arthritis, Parkinson's disease, or heart disease, engaging in physical activity may seem daunting or even impossible. However, with the right adaptations and guidance, these individuals can still reap the benefits of an active lifestyle.

By working closely with healthcare providers, physical therapists, or exercise specialists, older adults can develop a tailored exercise program that takes their specific limitations and needs into account. This may involve low-impact activities, seated exercises, or the use of assistive devices, all of which can help to safely and effectively improve physical function, reduce symptoms, and enhance overall well-being.

Fear of Injury or Falling

One of the primary concerns for older adults when it comes to physical activity is the fear of injury or falling. This apprehension is understandable, as the risk of falls and related injuries does increase with age. However, maintaining an active lifestyle can actually help to reduce the risk of falls by improving strength, balance, and coordination.

To address this concern, older adults can focus on incorporating balance-enhancing exercises, such as tai chi or Pilates, into their fitness routine. They can also work with a physical therapist or personal trainer to learn proper techniques and gradually build up their confidence and stability. Additionally, ensuring a safe and supportive environment, such as well-lit and obstacle-free spaces, can help to alleviate fears and encourage regular physical activity.

Lack of Motivation or Enjoyment

For some older adults, the idea of exercise can be daunting or simply not enjoyable, leading to a lack of motivation to maintain a consistent fitness routine. This can be particularly challenging for individuals who have been sedentary for a long time or who may not have found physical activities that they truly enjoy.

To overcome this barrier, it's important to explore a variety of physical activities and find ones that align with your personal interests and preferences. This may involve trying new sports, classes, or hobbies that you've never considered before, or revisiting activities you enjoyed in the past. Additionally, setting achievable goals, tracking your progress, and celebrating your successes can help to boost your motivation and make exercise a more rewarding experience.

Time Constraints and Competing Priorities

As we age, our schedules and priorities can often become more complex, with responsibilities such as caregiving, volunteer work, or part-time employment competing for our time and attention. In such cases, it can be challenging to carve out dedicated time for physical activity.

To address this barrier, it's important to be creative and find ways to integrate physical activity into your daily routine, as mentioned earlier. This could involve taking walking breaks during the workday, doing light exercises while watching TV, or combining physical activity with social engagements, such as going for a stroll with friends.

Additionally, older adults can explore shorter, high-intensity workouts or bodyweight exercises that can be performed at home, allowing them to fit physical activity into their schedules more easily.

Embracing the Transformative Power of Physical Activity

As we have explored in this chapter, regular physical activity and exercise are essential for maintaining physical, mental, and emotional well-being as we age. By incorporating a well-rounded fitness regimen into our daily lives, we can preserve our independence, reduce the risk of chronic diseases, and enhance our overall quality of life.

Whether it's strength training to maintain muscle mass, cardiovascular exercises to support heart health, or flexibility and balance activities to improve mobility, there are a myriad of ways for older adults to stay physically active and engaged. And by finding activities that we genuinely enjoy, and adapting our exercise routines as needed, we can make physical activity a sustainable and rewarding part of our daily lives.

Remember, the key to a successful and transformative fitness journey is to start small, be patient, and celebrate every step of progress. By embracing the power of physical activity and exercise, we can unlock a world of benefits that will enrich our golden years and beyond.

So, let's embark on this journey together, discovering new ways to move, challenge ourselves, and feel the incredible benefits of an active lifestyle. With determination, creativity, and a willingness to adapt, we can redefine the aging experience and unlock the boundless potential that lies within us. Get ready to feel stronger, more resilient, and more connected to your body and mind than ever before.

CHAPTER 4

Chapter 4: Cognitive Health and Brain Fitness

As we navigate the journey of healthy aging, one of the most crucial aspects we must address is the preservation and enhancement of our cognitive health. The ability to think clearly, remember important information, and adapt to new situations is not only essential for maintaining our independence and quality of life, but it also allows us to continue contributing to our communities and pursuing our passions well into our golden years.

In this chapter, we will delve into the science behind cognitive health and brain fitness, exploring the various factors that can impact our cognitive abilities as we age. We will then dive into a comprehensive toolkit of strategies and activities that can help you maintain and even improve your mental sharpness, problem-solving skills, and overall brain function.

By the end of this chapter, you will be armed with the knowledge and practical tools to embark on a transformative journey of brain health and cognitive rejuvenation, setting the stage for a fulfilling and mentally vibrant future.

Understanding Cognitive Health and the Aging Brain

As we grow older, our brains naturally undergo a series of changes, both in structure and function. While some cognitive decline is a normal part of the aging process, the rate and extent of these changes can be significantly influenced by our lifestyle choices, physical health, and overall well-being.

The Aging Brain: Neuroplasticity and Cognitive Decline

One of the key concepts in understanding cognitive health and the aging brain is neuroplasticity – the brain's remarkable ability to adapt, change, and reorganize itself in response to various stimuli and experiences. Throughout our lives, our brains are constantly rewiring and forming new neural connections, a process that allows us to learn, remember, and adapt to our environments.

However, as we age, the brain's neuroplasticity can begin to slow down, leading to a gradual decline in certain cognitive functions, such as processing speed, memory, and executive function (the skills needed for planning, decision-making, and problem-solving).

This age-related cognitive decline is a natural phenomenon, but the rate at which it occurs can be influenced by a variety of factors, including:

- Physical health and lifestyle: Conditions like cardiovascular disease, diabetes, and physical inactivity can accelerate cognitive decline.
    - Mental stimulation and engagement: Regularly challenging the brain through learning, problem-solving, and other cognitive exercises can help maintain and even improve cognitive abilities.
    - Stress and emotional well-being: Chronic stress and poor emotional health can negatively impact cognitive function.
    - Genetic and environmental factors: Certain genetic predispositions and exposure to environmental toxins may increase the risk of cognitive decline.

By understanding the factors that can influence cognitive health, we can take proactive steps to maintain and enhance our brain function as we age.

The Spectrum of Cognitive Decline

It's important to note that cognitive decline exists on a spectrum, ranging from normal age-related changes to more severe forms of cognitive impairment, such as mild cognitive impairment (MCI) and dementia, including Alzheimer's disease.

- Normal age-related cognitive changes: These are the gradual, expected declines in certain cognitive abilities that occur as a natural part of the aging process, such as slower processing speed or minor memory lapses.
  - Mild cognitive impairment (MCI): MCI represents a stage of cognitive decline that is more pronounced than normal age-related changes but does not significantly interfere with daily life. Individuals with MCI have an increased risk of developing dementia.
  - Dementia: Dementia is a term used to describe a more severe and debilitating form of cognitive decline that significantly impairs a person's ability to function independently. Alzheimer's disease is the most common type of dementia.

While the prospect of cognitive decline can be concerning, it's important to remember that the brain's remarkable neuroplasticity means that we have the power to influence our cognitive health and potentially slow or even reverse the effects of aging on our mental faculties.

Strategies for Maintaining and Enhancing Cognitive Health

By adopting a comprehensive, evidence-based approach to cognitive health, older adults can take proactive steps to maintain and even improve their mental sharpness, problem-solving abilities, and overall brain function. This multifaceted approach should encompass physical activity, mental stimulation, social engagement, and stress management – all of which have been shown to have a positive impact on cognitive function.

Physical Activity and Exercise

Regular physical activity has been consistently linked to improved cognitive function and a reduced risk of cognitive decline and dementia. Exercise can benefit the brain in several ways, including:

- Increasing blood flow and oxygen delivery to the brain
    - Stimulating the release of neurotransmitters and growth factors that support neuroplasticity
    - Reducing inflammation and oxidative stress, which can contribute to cognitive decline
    - Improving cardiovascular health, which is closely tied to brain health

Older adults should aim to incorporate a variety of physical activities into their routine, such as aerobic exercise (e.g., brisk walking, swimming, cycling), strength training, and flexibility exercises. By combining these different types of physical activity, older adults can optimize the benefits for their overall cognitive health.

Mental Stimulation and Cognitive Training

Just as physical exercise is important for the body, challenging the brain through cognitive activities and mental stimulation is crucial for maintaining and enhancing cognitive function. Engaging in a variety of mentally stimulating tasks can help build new neural connections, improve memory and problem-solving skills, and potentially delay the onset of cognitive decline.

Some effective strategies for mental stimulation and cognitive training include:

- Learning new skills, such as playing a musical instrument, mastering a new language, or taking up a new hobby

- Engaging in puzzles, brain teasers, and other cognitive challenges
- Participating in educational classes, lectures, or online courses
- Reading diverse materials, such as books, articles, and audiobooks
- Playing strategic games, such as chess, bridge, or sudoku

By regularly challenging the brain with a diverse range of cognitive activities, older adults can help maintain and potentially improve their mental acuity, problem-solving abilities, and overall cognitive function.

Social Engagement and Lifelong Learning

In addition to physical activity and cognitive training, social engagement and lifelong learning have also been shown to have a positive impact on cognitive health. Maintaining strong social connections and continuously seeking out new learning opportunities can help protect the brain against age-related decline.

Engaging in social activities, such as joining a club, volunteering, or participating in group classes or discussions, can provide cognitive benefits by:

- Stimulating the brain through social interaction and problem-solving
- Reducing the risk of social isolation and loneliness, which have been linked to cognitive decline
- Promoting a sense of purpose and belonging, which can positively impact emotional well-being

Similarly, embracing lifelong learning and continuously challenging the brain with new information and skills can help maintain and enhance cognitive function. Older adults can pursue this through formal education, such as taking college courses or attending adult learning programs, or through more informal means, such as reading, taking online classes, or attending lectures and workshops.

By actively engaging in social activities and maintaining a curious, lifelong learning mindset, older adults can support their cognitive health and overall well-being.

Stress Management and Emotional Well-being

Chronic stress and poor emotional health can have a significant impact on cognitive function, as they can contribute to inflammation, neuronal damage, and impaired neuroplasticity. Therefore, incorporating strategies for stress management and emotional well-being is an important component of a comprehensive approach to cognitive health.

Some effective stress management and emotional well-being strategies for older adults include:

- Practicing mindfulness, meditation, or other relaxation techniques
  - Engaging in regular exercise, which can help alleviate stress and improve mood
  - Developing a strong social support network and engaging in meaningful social activities
  - Seeking professional help, such as therapy or counseling, if needed
  - Prioritizing self-care activities, such as adequate sleep, a healthy diet, and regular leisure time

By addressing the emotional and psychological factors that can influence cognitive function, older adults can create a holistic foundation for maintaining and enhancing their mental abilities.

Dietary Considerations for Cognitive Health

The foods we consume can also play a crucial role in supporting cognitive function and brain health as we age. A balanced, nutrient-rich diet can provide the necessary building blocks for a healthy brain, while certain dietary patterns and specific nutrients have been linked to improved cognitive outcomes.

Some key dietary considerations for cognitive health include:

- Omega-3 fatty acids: Found in fatty fish, such as salmon and mackerel, as well as in walnuts and flaxseeds, omega-3s have been shown to support brain function and reduce the risk of cognitive decline.
- Antioxidants: Fruits, vegetables, and other plant-based foods rich in antioxidants, such as berries, leafy greens, and turmeric, can help protect the brain from oxidative stress and inflammation.
- B vitamins: Vitamins B6, B12, and folate play important roles in brain health and cognitive function, and may be particularly important for older adults.
- Mediterranean-style diet: This dietary pattern, characterized by a focus on plant-based foods, healthy fats, and limited processed items, has been associated with a reduced risk of cognitive decline and dementia.

By incorporating a nutrient-dense, brain-healthy diet into their overall lifestyle, older adults can further support their cognitive abilities and overall brain function.

Adapting Cognitive Health Strategies for Varying Needs

While the strategies outlined above can benefit the cognitive health of older adults in general, it's important to recognize that individual needs and abilities may vary. Some older adults may face specific challenges or limitations that require more tailored approaches to maintaining and enhancing their brain fitness.

Addressing Mild Cognitive Impairment (MCI)

For older adults who have been diagnosed with mild cognitive impairment

(MCI), a more targeted approach to cognitive health may be necessary. MCI represents a stage of cognitive decline that is more pronounced than normal age-related changes, but does not significantly interfere with daily life.

In addition to the general strategies for cognitive health, individuals with MCI may benefit from:

- Cognitive rehabilitation or training programs specifically designed for MCI
   - Occupational therapy to develop compensatory strategies for cognitive challenges
   - Regular monitoring and assessments by healthcare professionals to track progress
   - Addressing any underlying medical conditions that may be contributing to MCI

By addressing the specific needs and challenges associated with MCI, older adults can work to maintain their cognitive function, slow the progression of decline, and potentially even reverse some of the symptoms.

Considerations for Those with Dementia or Alzheimer's Disease

For older adults living with more severe forms of cognitive decline, such as dementia or Alzheimer's disease, the approach to cognitive health must be adapted to their unique needs and abilities. While the general strategies can still be beneficial, the implementation and focus may need to be adjusted.

Some key considerations for those with dementia or Alzheimer's include:

- Tailoring cognitive activities and mental stimulation to their current level of function and attention span
   - Incorporating sensory-based activities, such as music, art, or aromatherapy, to engage the brain in different ways
   - Prioritizing safety, routine, and environmental modifications to support

daily functioning
  - Involving caregivers and loved ones in the care and support plan
  - Seeking guidance from healthcare professionals, such as geriatric psychiatrists or dementia care specialists

By taking a personalized and adaptable approach to cognitive health, individuals with more advanced cognitive decline can still benefit from interventions that support their brain function, maintain their quality of life, and provide comfort and support for both the individual and their caregivers.

Embracing the Journey of Cognitive Rejuvenation

As we have explored in this chapter, maintaining and enhancing cognitive health is a critical component of healthy aging. By adopting a comprehensive, evidence-based approach that encompasses physical activity, mental stimulation, social engagement, and emotional well-being, older adults can take proactive steps to preserve their cognitive abilities and potentially even improve their mental faculties.

Remember, the aging brain is a remarkable and dynamic organ, constantly adapting and reorganizing itself in response to our experiences and lifestyle choices. By regularly challenging ourselves, staying socially and intellectually engaged, and managing stress and emotional well-being, we can harness the brain's remarkable neuroplasticity and unlock its full potential.

As you embark on this journey of cognitive rejuvenation, be patient, persistent, and open to trying new activities and strategies. What works for one individual may not be the best fit for another, so be willing to experiment and find the approaches that resonate most with you. Celebrate your successes, no matter how small, and don't be discouraged by any setbacks – the brain is resilient, and with consistent effort, you can continue to grow and thrive.

Ultimately, the path to cognitive health is a lifelong journey, one that requires a holistic and adaptable approach. By prioritizing your brain fitness, you are not only investing in your own well-being but also setting an inspiring example for those around you. Together, let's redefine the narrative of aging and demonstrate the boundless potential of the human mind.

CHAPTER 5

Chapter 5: Emotional Well-being and Stress Management

As we navigate the journey of healthy aging, it's essential to recognize that our physical health and cognitive abilities are intrinsically linked to our emotional well-being. The way we manage stress, cultivate positive emotions, and maintain strong social connections can have a profound impact on our overall quality of life and our ability to thrive in the golden years.

In this chapter, we will delve into the critical role of emotional well-being and stress management in the context of healthy aging. We will explore the various factors that can influence our emotional state, the importance of fostering social connections, and proven strategies for reducing stress and anxiety. By the end of this chapter, you will be equipped with the knowledge and tools to nurture your emotional resilience, enhance your mental and physical health, and create a fulfilling, balanced lifestyle in the years to come.

The Importance of Emotional Well-being in Healthy Aging

Emotional well-being is a multifaceted concept that encompasses our ability to manage our feelings, maintain positive relationships, and find meaning and purpose in our lives. As we grow older, the preservation and enhancement of our emotional well-being become increasingly crucial, as it can have a significant impact on our overall health, cognitive function, and quality of life.

The Link Between Emotional and Physical Health

The relationship between our emotional and physical health is deeply intertwined. Chronic stress, depression, and anxiety can take a toll on our bodies, contributing to a range of health issues, including cardiovascular disease, weakened immune function, and increased inflammation.

Conversely, physical health challenges, such as chronic pain, disability, or chronic illness, can also have a profound impact on our emotional well-being, leading to feelings of frustration, isolation, and even depression. By addressing both the emotional and physical aspects of our health, we can create a positive feedback loop that enhances our overall well-being and resilience.

The Cognitive Benefits of Emotional Well-being

Emotional well-being and cognitive health are also closely linked. Positive emotions, such as joy, gratitude, and a sense of purpose, can support neuroplasticity, the brain's ability to adapt and change over time. This, in turn, can improve memory, problem-solving skills, and overall cognitive function.

Conversely, chronic stress and negative emotions, such as anxiety and depression, can have a detrimental impact on the brain, contributing to impaired memory, reduced cognitive flexibility, and an increased risk of dementia. By prioritizing emotional well-being, older adults can help maintain and even enhance their cognitive abilities, enabling them to continue learning, problem-solving, and engaging in intellectually stimulating activities.

The Importance of Social Connections

One of the key components of emotional well-being is the presence of strong, meaningful social connections. As we age, maintaining a robust social support network can have a profound impact on our mental health, physical health, and overall quality of life.

Positive social interactions and a sense of belonging can help reduce feelings of loneliness and isolation, which are common challenges for older adults. Moreover, engaging in social activities can provide a sense of purpose, foster a positive emotional state, and even contribute to better cognitive function.

Conversely, social isolation and loneliness have been linked to a range of negative health outcomes, including depression, cardiovascular disease, and even increased mortality. By prioritizing social engagement and cultivating meaningful relationships, older adults can enhance their emotional well-being and support their overall health and resilience.

Strategies for Enhancing Emotional Well-being

Given the critical importance of emotional well-being in the context of healthy aging, it's essential to incorporate a comprehensive, evidence-based approach to nurturing our mental and emotional health. This multi-faceted strategy should include a combination of self-care practices, stress management techniques, and strategies for fostering social connections.

Practicing Self-care and Mindfulness

One of the fundamental pillars of emotional well-being is the incorporation of self-care practices into our daily routines. Self-care can take many forms, from engaging in relaxing activities to prioritizing our physical and mental health needs.

Mindfulness, a practice that involves being present in the moment and cultivating a non-judgmental awareness of our thoughts, emotions, and physical sensations, can be particularly beneficial for older adults. Regular mindfulness practice has been shown to reduce stress, improve emotional regulation, and enhance overall well-being.

Some effective self-care and mindfulness strategies for older adults include:

- Engaging in relaxation techniques, such as deep breathing, meditation, or progressive muscle relaxation
   - Incorporating gentle physical activities, such as yoga, tai chi, or leisurely walks
   - Pursuing hobbies and creative activities that bring a sense of joy and purpose
   - Practicing gratitude, either through journaling or sharing appreciations with others
   - Prioritizing adequate sleep and rest to support physical and emotional restoration

By making self-care and mindfulness a regular part of their routine, older adults can nourish their emotional well-being, manage stress, and enhance their overall quality of life.

Managing Stress and Anxiety

Chronic stress and anxiety can have a significant impact on our emotional, cognitive, and physical health, making it essential to develop effective strategies for managing these challenging emotions. Older adults may face a range of stressors, from health concerns and financial worries to the loss of loved ones and the adjustments of retirement.

By incorporating stress management techniques into their daily lives, older adults can learn to better cope with these challenges and maintain a sense of emotional balance and resilience. Some effective strategies include:

- Practicing relaxation techniques, such as deep breathing, meditation, or progressive muscle relaxation
    - Engaging in regular physical activity, which can help alleviate the physical and emotional symptoms of stress
    - Seeking support from friends, family, or mental health professionals, such as therapists or counselors
    - Developing healthy coping mechanisms, such as journaling, engaging in hobbies, or practicing mindfulness
    - Prioritizing self-care activities, such as getting enough sleep, eating a balanced diet, and taking breaks from stressful situations

By addressing stress and anxiety proactively, older adults can enhance their emotional well-being, improve their cognitive function, and support their overall physical health.

Fostering Social Connections and Relationships

As previously mentioned, maintaining a strong social support network is essential for emotional well-being in the context of healthy aging. However, as we grow older, we may face challenges in cultivating and sustaining these meaningful connections, such as the loss of friends and loved ones, retirement, or reduced mobility.

To combat social isolation and foster a sense of belonging, older adults can engage in a variety of strategies, such as:

- Joining social clubs, hobby groups, or community organizations that align with their interests
    - Participating in volunteer work or giving back to their communities
    - Regularly connecting with friends and family, either in person or through virtual means
    - Exploring opportunities for intergenerational connections, such as mentoring younger individuals or engaging with grandchildren

- Seeking out support groups or social activities specifically designed for older adults

By actively cultivating and nurturing their social connections, older adults can enhance their emotional well-being, reduce feelings of loneliness and isolation, and maintain a strong sense of purpose and belonging.

Addressing Specific Emotional Health Challenges

While the strategies outlined above can benefit the emotional well-being of older adults in general, it's important to recognize that individuals may face specific emotional health challenges that require more tailored approaches. By addressing these challenges proactively, older adults can improve their overall quality of life and maintain their resilience in the face of adversity.

Managing Depression and Anxiety

Depression and anxiety are common emotional health challenges for older adults, and they can have a significant impact on their physical health, cognitive function, and overall quality of life. Factors such as chronic health conditions, social isolation, and the loss of loved ones can all contribute to the development of these mental health issues.

To address depression and anxiety, older adults can incorporate a combination of therapeutic interventions, lifestyle modifications, and social support. Some effective strategies include:

- Seeking professional help from a mental health provider, such as a therapist or counselor, who can develop a personalized treatment plan
    - Engaging in regular exercise, which has been shown to have a positive impact on mood and anxiety levels
    - Practicing relaxation techniques, such as meditation, deep breathing, or guided imagery

- Cultivating a strong social support network and engaging in activities that foster a sense of purpose and meaning
- Exploring the use of cognitive-behavioral therapy (CBT) or other evidence-based therapeutic approaches

By addressing depression and anxiety proactively, older adults can improve their emotional well-being, enhance their physical health, and maintain their independence and quality of life.

Coping with Grief and Loss

Older adults often face the challenge of dealing with the loss of loved ones, whether through death, relocation, or the natural progression of life. Grief and bereavement can be profoundly difficult to navigate, and they can have a significant impact on emotional well-being.

To support older adults in coping with grief and loss, it's important to:

- Allow time and space for the grieving process, recognizing that it is a unique and personal experience
- Encourage the individual to share their feelings and memories with trusted friends or family members
- Suggest participation in support groups or grief counseling, which can provide a safe space for expression and healing
- Recommend the use of coping strategies, such as journaling, creating a memorial, or engaging in activities that were meaningful to the lost loved one
- Remind the individual that it's important to be patient and gentle with themselves, as the grieving process can be unpredictable and long-lasting

By providing compassionate support and guidance, older adults can navigate the complex emotions of grief and loss, find ways to honor their loved ones, and ultimately integrate the experience into their lives in a healthy and meaningful way.

Addressing Caregiver Burnout

For older adults who find themselves in the role of caregiver for a spouse, family member, or friend, the emotional and physical demands of this responsibility can lead to a condition known as caregiver burnout. This state of physical, emotional, and mental exhaustion can have a significant impact on the caregiver's well-being and their ability to provide effective care.

To address caregiver burnout, it's essential for older adults to prioritize their own self-care and seek support from others. Strategies may include:

- Regularly scheduling breaks and respite care to allow the caregiver time to rest and recharge
    - Joining a support group for caregivers, where they can share experiences and coping strategies
    - Enlisting the help of family members, friends, or professional caregivers to share the responsibilities
    - Incorporating stress management techniques, such as relaxation exercises or mindfulness practices, into their daily routine
    - Seeking counseling or therapy to process the emotional challenges of caregiving

By addressing caregiver burnout proactively, older adults can maintain their own emotional well-being, enhance their ability to provide care, and ultimately improve the quality of life for both themselves and the individual they are caring for.

Embracing a Holistic Approach to Emotional Well-being

Emotional well-being is a multifaceted and dynamic aspect of healthy aging, and it requires a comprehensive, holistic approach to nurture and maintain. By integrating the various strategies and techniques outlined in this chapter, older adults can create a supportive and resilient foundation for their emotional health, ultimately enhancing their overall quality of life.

Remember, emotional well-being is not a static state, but rather a continuous journey of self-discovery, adaptability, and growth. As we navigate the challenges and transitions of aging, it's essential to remain open, flexible, and willing to try new approaches to managing our emotions and fostering meaningful connections.

Moreover, embracing emotional well-being is not just about individual benefits – it can also have a profound impact on our communities and the broader society. By sharing our experiences, providing support to others, and setting an example of emotional resilience, older adults can inspire and empower those around them, creating a ripple effect of well-being that benefits people of all ages.

As you embark on this journey of emotional rejuvenation, be patient, compassionate, and willing to seek support when needed. Remember that emotional well-being is not a solitary pursuit, but rather a collaborative effort that involves friends, family, and healthcare professionals. By fostering a strong support network and continuously exploring new ways to nurture your emotional health, you can unlock a world of possibilities and create a fulfilling, balanced life in the golden years and beyond.

CHAPTER 6

Chapter 6: Sleep and Healthy Aging

As we embark on the journey of healthy aging, one of the often-overlooked, yet critically important, aspects of our well-being is the quality and quantity of our sleep. Sleep plays a vital role in supporting physical health, cognitive function, and emotional well-being, all of which are essential for maintaining independence, resilience, and a high quality of life as we grow older.

In this chapter, we will explore the unique sleep-related challenges and considerations that often accompany the aging process, and we will delve into a comprehensive toolkit of strategies and solutions to help you optimize your sleep and reap the multifaceted benefits of quality rest.

The Importance of Sleep in Healthy Aging

Sleep is a fundamental biological necessity, a restorative process that allows our bodies and minds to recharge, repair, and rejuvenate. However, as we age, we often experience significant changes in our sleep patterns and quality, which can have far-reaching implications for our overall health and well-being.

The Impact of Sleep on Physical Health

Adequate, high-quality sleep is essential for maintaining optimal physical health as we grow older. During sleep, our bodies undergo crucial restorative processes, such as tissue repair, immune function enhancement, and hormone regulation – all of which are vital for preventing age-related diseases and maintaining physical vitality.

Conversely, chronic sleep deprivation or poor sleep quality has been linked to an increased risk of a variety of health issues, including:

- Cardiovascular disease: Lack of sleep can contribute to high blood pressure, heart disease, and stroke.
- Metabolic disorders: Sleep disturbances can disrupt blood sugar regulation and increase the risk of type 2 diabetes.
- Weakened immune system: Poor sleep can impair the body's ability to fight off infections and illnesses.
- Increased inflammation: Chronic sleep loss is associated with higher levels of inflammatory markers, which can accelerate the aging process.

By prioritizing quality sleep and addressing any underlying sleep-related challenges, older adults can support their physical health, reduce the risk of age-related diseases, and maintain their independence and overall well-being.

The Impact of Sleep on Cognitive Function

In addition to its physical health benefits, quality sleep also plays a critical role in maintaining and enhancing cognitive function as we age. During sleep, our brains undergo essential processes, such as memory consolidation, neural plasticity, and the clearing of metabolic waste – all of which are crucial for preserving cognitive abilities, including learning, memory, and problem-solving skills.

Conversely, chronic sleep disturbances have been linked to a range of cognitive impairments, including:

- Decreased memory and recall: Lack of sleep can impair the brain's ability to consolidate and retrieve memories.
  - Reduced attention and focus: Poor sleep quality can make it more difficult to concentrate and pay attention.
  - Diminished problem-solving and decision-making skills: Sleep deprivation can negatively impact executive function and the brain's ability to process information.
  - Increased risk of dementia: Disrupted sleep patterns have been associated with a higher risk of developing Alzheimer's disease and other forms of dementia.

By ensuring adequate, high-quality sleep, older adults can support their cognitive health, maintain their mental sharpness, and potentially delay or even prevent age-related cognitive decline.

The Impact of Sleep on Emotional Well-being

The relationship between sleep and emotional well-being is a complex and reciprocal one. On the one hand, poor sleep can contribute to increased stress, anxiety, and depression, which can, in turn, further disrupt sleep patterns. On the other hand, maintaining healthy sleep habits can support emotional regulation, improve mood, and enhance overall psychological resilience.

Chronic sleep disturbances have been linked to a range of emotional health challenges, including:

- Increased risk of depression and anxiety: Lack of sleep can contribute to the development and exacerbation of these mental health conditions.
  - Decreased emotional regulation: Poor sleep can make it more difficult to manage and express emotions in a healthy, constructive manner.
  - Reduced social engagement and quality of life: Sleep-related issues can lead to feelings of fatigue, irritability, and social withdrawal.

By prioritizing quality sleep and addressing any underlying sleep-related challenges, older adults can support their emotional well-being, enhance their ability to cope with stress and life transitions, and maintain a positive, resilient outlook on the aging process.

Understanding Age-related Changes in Sleep Patterns

As we grow older, our sleep patterns and sleep quality often undergo significant changes, which can be influenced by a variety of physiological, psychological, and environmental factors. Understanding these age-related sleep changes can help older adults develop more effective strategies for optimizing their sleep and addressing any sleep-related challenges.

Changes in Sleep Architecture

One of the primary changes that occurs in the sleep patterns of older adults is a shift in sleep architecture, or the structure and organization of the different stages of sleep. As we age, we tend to experience:

- Reduced total sleep time: Older adults often sleep fewer hours than younger individuals, with an average of 6-7 hours of sleep per night.
  - Increased light sleep and reduced deep sleep: The time spent in deep, restorative sleep (known as slow-wave sleep) decreases, while the amount of light, fragmented sleep increases.
  - More frequent nighttime awakenings: Older adults often experience more interruptions in their sleep, leading to reduced sleep continuity and quality.

These changes in sleep architecture can contribute to feelings of non-restorative sleep, daytime fatigue, and an increased susceptibility to sleep-related health issues.

Circadian Rhythm Shifts

In addition to changes in sleep architecture, the aging process can also lead to shifts in the body's circadian rhythms, the internal 24-hour clock that regulates our sleep-wake cycles and other physiological processes.

As we grow older, the body's natural circadian rhythms can become less synchronized, leading to:

- Earlier bedtimes and wake times: Older adults often go to bed and wake up earlier than they did in their younger years.
    - Increased daytime sleepiness: The changes in circadian rhythms can cause older adults to feel more tired during the day, leading to napping or dozing off.
    - Difficulty falling and staying asleep: Disruptions to the body's internal clock can make it harder for older adults to initiate and maintain sleep.

These circadian rhythm shifts can further contribute to the sleep challenges faced by older adults and may require targeted interventions to help reestablish a healthy sleep-wake cycle.

Common Sleep Disorders in Older Adults

In addition to the age-related changes in sleep patterns, older adults may also be more susceptible to certain sleep disorders, which can significantly impact their overall health and well-being. Some of the most common sleep disorders in this population include:

- Insomnia: Difficulty falling asleep, staying asleep, or obtaining restorative sleep, which can be exacerbated by factors such as chronic health conditions, medications, or stress.
    - Sleep apnea: A disorder characterized by repeated breathing interruptions during sleep, leading to fragmented sleep and decreased oxygen levels.
    - Restless Leg Syndrome (RLS): A neurological condition that causes an irresistible urge to move the legs, often resulting in disrupted sleep.

- Rapid Eye Movement (REM) Sleep Behavior Disorder: A condition in which individuals act out their dreams, potentially leading to injury or sleep disturbances.

By understanding the various sleep-related changes and challenges that older adults may face, we can develop more targeted and effective strategies for optimizing sleep and supporting overall health and well-being.

Strategies for Improving Sleep in Older Adults

Fortunately, there are a variety of evidence-based strategies and interventions that older adults can implement to improve their sleep quality, address any underlying sleep-related issues, and reap the numerous benefits of quality rest. These strategies should be tailored to the individual's specific needs and circumstances, as the approach to sleep optimization may vary based on factors such as health status, lifestyle, and personal preferences.

Establishing Good Sleep Hygiene

One of the foundational elements of improving sleep quality for older adults is the adoption of good sleep hygiene practices. Sleep hygiene refers to the habits, environment, and behaviors that can either promote or hinder restful sleep. By incorporating the following sleep hygiene principles, older adults can create a supportive sleep environment and encourage better sleep quality:

- Maintain a consistent sleep-wake schedule, even on weekends or during retirement.
- Establish a relaxing pre-bedtime routine, such as taking a warm bath, reading a book, or engaging in light stretching.
- Ensure the sleeping environment is dark, cool, and quiet, with comfortable bedding and minimal distractions.
- Avoid or limit the use of electronic devices (e.g., phones, tablets, TVs) in the bedroom, as the blue light emitted by these devices can disrupt the body's

natural sleep-wake cycle.

 - Limit daytime napping, or ensure that naps are kept to a reasonable duration (e.g., 30 minutes or less).

 - Avoid consuming caffeine, alcohol, or heavy meals close to bedtime, as these can interfere with sleep quality.

By establishing and consistently following good sleep hygiene practices, older adults can create a foundation for improved sleep and better overall health.

Engaging in Regular Physical Activity

As discussed in previous chapters, regular physical activity and exercise play a crucial role in supporting healthy aging, and this includes the optimization of sleep quality. Engaging in various types of physical activity, such as aerobic exercise, strength training, or low-impact activities like walking or tai chi, can have a positive impact on sleep in several ways:

- Promoting better sleep onset and sleep efficiency by reducing the time it takes to fall asleep and increasing the amount of time spent in deep, restorative sleep.

 - Alleviating symptoms of certain sleep disorders, such as sleep apnea and restless leg syndrome, by improving cardiovascular health and reducing muscle tension.

 - Enhancing daytime alertness and energy levels, which can help older adults maintain a consistent sleep-wake cycle.

It's important to note that the timing and intensity of physical activity can also influence sleep, so older adults should aim to complete their workouts several hours before bedtime and avoid intense exercise close to bedtime, as this can have a stimulating effect and disrupt sleep.

Incorporating Relaxation Techniques

Stress and anxiety can be significant contributors to sleep disturbances in older adults, so incorporating relaxation techniques into one's daily routine can be a highly effective strategy for improving sleep quality. Some effective relaxation techniques include:

- Mindfulness meditation: Practicing focused attention on the breath, body, or present moment can help reduce stress and promote a calm, restful state.
- Progressive muscle relaxation: Systematically tensing and releasing different muscle groups to induce a state of physical and mental relaxation.
- Deep breathing exercises: Engaging in slow, deep breathing patterns to activate the parasympathetic nervous system and induce a sense of calm.
- Guided imagery or visualization: Imagining peaceful, calming scenes or scenarios to shift the mind away from sources of stress or worry.

By regularly practicing these relaxation techniques, older adults can better manage stress, improve their ability to fall and stay asleep, and enhance the overall quality of their sleep.

Addressing Underlying Health Conditions

In many cases, sleep disturbances in older adults may be linked to underlying health conditions, such as chronic pain, respiratory issues, or neurological disorders. It's essential for older adults to work closely with their healthcare providers to identify and address any underlying health concerns that may be contributing to their sleep problems.

Some common health conditions that can impact sleep in older adults include:

- Chronic pain (e.g., arthritis, neuropathy)
- Respiratory disorders (e.g., chronic obstructive pulmonary disease, sleep apnea)
- Neurological conditions (e.g., Parkinson's disease, Alzheimer's disease)
- Endocrine disorders (e.g., thyroid imbalances, diabetes)

By working with their healthcare team to properly manage these underlying conditions, older adults can often experience significant improvements in their sleep quality and overall well-being.

Considering Medication and Supplements

In some cases, older adults may benefit from the use of medication or dietary supplements to address specific sleep-related issues. However, it's crucial to consult with a healthcare provider before starting any new medications or supplements, as they can interact with existing medications or have other side effects, particularly in older individuals.

Some common sleep-related medications and supplements that may be considered for older adults include:

- Prescription sleep medications: Used judiciously and under medical supervision to address chronic insomnia.
  - Melatonin: A naturally occurring hormone that can help regulate the sleep-wake cycle.
  - Valerian root: A herbal supplement that may have mild sedative effects and improve sleep quality.
  - Magnesium: A mineral that plays a role in sleep-wake regulation and can help alleviate symptoms of certain sleep disorders.

It's important to note that the use of sleep medications and supplements should be approached with caution in older adults, as they may have increased sensitivity to the effects and a higher risk of adverse reactions.

Embracing the Transformative Power of Quality Sleep

As we have explored in this chapter, quality sleep is a fundamental pillar of healthy aging, with far-reaching implications for our physical health, cognitive function, and emotional well-being. By understanding the unique sleep-related challenges faced by older adults and implementing a comprehensive, evidence-based approach to sleep optimization, we can unlock a world of benefits and support our overall vitality and resilience.

Remember, the journey to better sleep is not a one-size-fits-all approach. Each individual may have unique needs, preferences, and circumstances that require a tailored strategy. By experimenting with different techniques, being patient and persistent, and seeking guidance from healthcare professionals when needed, older adults can find the sleep solutions that work best for them.

Investing in quality sleep is an investment in your overall health and well-being. By prioritizing sleep, you are not only supporting your immediate physical and mental state but also laying the groundwork for a more vibrant, independent, and fulfilling future. Embrace the transformative power of sleep, and embark on a journey of rejuvenation and vitality that will carry you through the golden years and beyond.

Remember, you are not alone in this pursuit. Reach out to your healthcare providers, support networks, and the wider community of older adults who are committed to optimizing their sleep and overall health. Together, we can create a culture of healthy aging that celebrates the importance of quality rest and its profound impact on our lives.

So, let's dive in, explore the sleep-related strategies that resonate most with you, and unlock the boundless potential that awaits when we prioritize our sleep and overall well-being. The future is bright, and it starts with a good night's rest.

CHAPTER 7

hapter 7: Chronic Disease Prevention and Management

As we navigate the journey of healthy aging, one of the most crucial aspects of maintaining our well-being is the prevention and management of chronic diseases. These persistent, long-term conditions can have a significant impact on our physical health, cognitive function, and overall quality of life, making them a critical consideration for older adults.

In this chapter, we will explore the landscape of common age-related chronic diseases, delving into the risk factors, prevention strategies, and effective management approaches. By understanding the science behind these conditions and the proactive steps we can take to address them, we can empower ourselves to take control of our health and create a fulfilling, independent, and resilient future.

Understanding Common Age-related Chronic Diseases

As we grow older, the risk of developing various chronic health conditions increases, often due to a combination of genetic, lifestyle, and environmental factors. While some of these conditions are more common in older adults, it's essential to recognize that the onset and progression of many chronic diseases can be significantly influenced by the choices we make throughout our lives.

Cardiovascular Disease

Cardiovascular disease, which encompasses conditions such as heart disease, stroke, and high blood pressure, is one of the leading causes of morbidity and mortality among older adults. Factors that can increase the risk of cardiovascular disease include:

- High blood pressure (hypertension)
    - High cholesterol levels
    - Diabetes and insulin resistance
    - Sedentary lifestyle and physical inactivity
    - Unhealthy dietary habits, such as a diet high in saturated and trans fats
    - Smoking and excessive alcohol consumption

By adopting a heart-healthy lifestyle, which includes regular exercise, a balanced diet, and the management of underlying risk factors, older adults can significantly reduce their risk of developing cardiovascular disease and its associated complications.

Type 2 Diabetes

Type 2 diabetes is another highly prevalent chronic condition among older adults, characterized by the body's inability to effectively regulate blood sugar levels. Factors that can contribute to the development of type 2 diabetes include:

- Excess body weight, particularly in the abdominal area
    - Sedentary lifestyle and physical inactivity
    - Unhealthy dietary habits, such as a diet high in refined carbohydrates and added sugars
    - Genetic predisposition and family history

Proactive management of type 2 diabetes, through a combination of lifestyle modifications, medication (if necessary), and regular monitoring, can help older adults maintain stable blood sugar levels, prevent or delay the onset of complications, and improve their overall health and well-being.

Arthritis

Arthritis, a group of conditions characterized by joint inflammation and pain, is another common chronic health concern for older adults. The two most prevalent forms of arthritis are osteoarthritis and rheumatoid arthritis. Factors that can contribute to the development of arthritis include:

- Age-related wear and tear on the joints
    - Genetic predisposition
    - Excess body weight, which can put additional stress on the joints
    - Past injuries or trauma to the joints
    - Autoimmune dysfunction (in the case of rheumatoid arthritis)

By adopting strategies to maintain joint health, such as regular exercise, weight management, and the use of assistive devices when needed, older adults can manage the symptoms of arthritis and maintain their mobility and independence.

Cognitive Decline and Dementia

As discussed in a previous chapter, cognitive decline and the development of dementia, such as Alzheimer's disease, are significant health concerns for older adults. While some degree of age-related cognitive change is normal, factors that can increase the risk of more severe cognitive impairment include:

- Cardiovascular disease and related risk factors
    - Traumatic brain injuries
    - Chronic stress and depression

- Sedentary lifestyle and physical inactivity
- Certain dietary and lifestyle factors, such as a poor-quality diet and excessive alcohol consumption

By adopting a comprehensive, evidence-based approach to brain health, including regular physical activity, cognitive stimulation, and the management of underlying health conditions, older adults can help reduce the risk of cognitive decline and maintain their mental acuity.

Cancer

Cancer is another chronic condition that becomes more prevalent with age, with the risk of developing certain types of cancer increasing significantly after the age of 65. Factors that can influence the risk of cancer in older adults include:

- Genetic predisposition and family history
- Lifestyle factors, such as smoking, excessive alcohol consumption, and poor dietary habits
- Environmental exposures, such as ultraviolet radiation or toxic substances
- Weakened immune system and impaired cellular repair mechanisms

While the risk of cancer increases with age, regular cancer screenings, a healthy lifestyle, and proactive management of any diagnosed cancers can greatly improve outcomes and quality of life for older adults.

Adopting a Proactive Approach to Chronic Disease Prevention

The prevention of chronic diseases is a crucial aspect of healthy aging, as it can help older adults maintain their independence, reduce the burden on healthcare systems, and enhance their overall quality of life. By adopting a proactive, comprehensive approach to chronic disease prevention, older adults can take control of their health and create a more vibrant, resilient future.

Maintaining a Healthy Lifestyle

One of the most effective ways to prevent the development of chronic diseases is by adopting a healthy lifestyle. This includes:

- Engaging in regular physical activity, as discussed in a previous chapter
    - Maintaining a balanced, nutrient-dense diet that emphasizes whole, unprocessed foods
    - Avoiding or limiting the use of tobacco products and excessive alcohol consumption
    - Prioritizing stress management and emotional well-being
    - Ensuring adequate sleep and rest

By making these healthy lifestyle choices a consistent part of their daily routines, older adults can significantly reduce their risk of developing a wide range of chronic conditions, from cardiovascular disease to cancer.

Managing Underlying Health Conditions

For older adults who may already have one or more chronic health conditions, such as hypertension or diabetes, it's essential to work closely with their healthcare providers to effectively manage these underlying issues. This may involve:

- Regularly monitoring and controlling risk factors, such as blood pressure, blood sugar levels, and cholesterol
    - Adhering to prescribed medications and treatment plans
    - Making necessary lifestyle modifications, such as adjusting dietary habits or increasing physical activity
    - Attending regular check-ups and screenings to detect any changes or complications early on

By proactively managing their underlying health conditions, older adults can help prevent the development of more severe chronic diseases and maintain their overall well-being.

Participating in Preventive Screenings

Regular preventive screenings and check-ups are another critical component of chronic disease prevention for older adults. These screenings can help detect the early signs of various health conditions, allowing for timely intervention and the implementation of effective management strategies.

Some common preventive screenings that older adults should consider include:

- Cancer screenings (e.g., mammograms, colonoscopies, prostate exams)
  - Cardiovascular health assessments (e.g., blood pressure checks, cholesterol tests)
  - Diabetes screening (e.g., fasting blood glucose, hemoglobin A1C tests)
  - Bone density scans to detect osteoporosis
  - Cognitive and neurological assessments

By staying up-to-date with these preventive screenings and working closely with their healthcare providers, older adults can proactively identify and address any emerging health concerns, reducing the risk of chronic disease progression and improving their overall health outcomes.

Incorporating Immunizations and Vaccinations

In addition to regular preventive screenings, older adults should also prioritize immunizations and vaccinations as a means of chronic disease prevention. As we age, our immune systems become less robust, making us more susceptible to certain infectious diseases that can lead to serious complications or chronic health issues.

Some key immunizations and vaccinations that older adults should consider include:

- Influenza (flu) vaccine: Helps prevent severe illness and complications from the flu
    - Pneumococcal vaccines: Protect against pneumonia, meningitis, and other pneumococcal diseases
    - Shingles vaccine: Reduces the risk of developing shingles, a painful viral infection
    - Tetanus, diphtheria, and pertussis (Tdap) vaccine: Helps maintain immunity against these serious bacterial infections

By staying up-to-date with these essential vaccinations, older adults can bolster their immune systems, reduce their susceptibility to infectious diseases, and prevent the development of chronic health issues that can arise from these illnesses.

Strategies for Managing Chronic Diseases

While prevention is a crucial aspect of healthy aging, there may be times when older adults are faced with the reality of managing one or more chronic health conditions. In these cases, it's essential to have a comprehensive, evidence-based approach to disease management that empowers older adults to take an active role in their care and maintain their quality of life.

Adopting a Multidisciplinary Approach

Effective chronic disease management often requires a multidisciplinary approach, involving a team of healthcare professionals who can address the various aspects of the condition and provide personalized, coordinated care. This team may include:

- Primary care physicians or geriatric specialists

- Specialists relevant to the specific chronic condition (e.g., cardiologists, endocrinologists, rheumatologists)
- Nurses and nurse practitioners
- Pharmacists
- Physical therapists, occupational therapists, and other rehabilitation specialists
- Mental health professionals, such as counselors or social workers

By working closely with this multidisciplinary team, older adults can develop a comprehensive care plan that addresses their physical, emotional, and social needs, empowering them to actively manage their chronic conditions and maintain their independence.

Developing Self-management Skills

In addition to working with a multidisciplinary healthcare team, older adults can also take an active role in managing their chronic conditions by developing essential self-management skills. This may include:

- Understanding the nature of their chronic condition, its symptoms, and the importance of treatment adherence
- Actively participating in the decision-making process regarding their care plan and treatment options
- Monitoring their own health metrics, such as blood pressure, blood sugar levels, or pain levels
- Incorporating lifestyle modifications, such as dietary changes or physical activity, into their daily routines
- Effectively communicating with their healthcare providers and advocating for their needs

By cultivating these self-management skills, older adults can become more empowered, engaged, and proactive in their care, leading to better health outcomes and a greater sense of control over their chronic conditions.

Utilizing Assistive Devices and Adaptive Technologies

As older adults navigate the challenges of chronic disease management, the use of assistive devices and adaptive technologies can play a crucial role in maintaining their independence and quality of life. These tools can help individuals adapt to physical limitations, improve mobility, and enhance their ability to perform everyday tasks.

Some examples of assistive devices and adaptive technologies for older adults with chronic conditions include:

- Mobility aids, such as walkers, canes, or wheelchairs
    - Home modifications, such as grab bars, ramps, or stair lifts
    - Durable medical equipment, such as oxygen tanks or continuous positive airway pressure (CPAP) machines
    - Telehealth and remote monitoring technologies to facilitate virtual healthcare visits and ongoing health tracking

By incorporating these assistive devices and adaptive technologies into their daily lives, older adults can overcome physical barriers, manage their chronic conditions more effectively, and continue to live independently and with a higher quality of life.

Accessing Community Resources and Support Services

Navigating the challenges of chronic disease management can be daunting, but older adults do not have to do it alone. By tapping into the various community resources and support services available, they can access additional assistance, education, and social connections that can enhance their overall well-being.

Some examples of community resources and support services for older adults with chronic conditions include:

- Chronic disease self-management programs and workshops
  - Support groups, either in-person or online, for specific chronic conditions
  - Meal delivery services or community meal programs
  - Transportation assistance for medical appointments or errands
  - In-home care services, such as nursing or personal care aides
  - Respite care services to provide temporary relief for caregivers

By actively seeking out and utilizing these community resources, older adults can supplement their healthcare team, expand their support network, and gain the necessary tools and knowledge to better manage their chronic conditions.

Embracing a Holistic Approach to Chronic Disease Prevention and Management

As we have explored in this chapter, the prevention and management of chronic diseases are critical components of healthy aging, with far-reaching implications for our physical, cognitive, and emotional well-being. By adopting a comprehensive, holistic approach that addresses the multifaceted nature of these conditions, older adults can take control of their health, reduce the burden of chronic diseases, and create a more vibrant, independent, and fulfilling future.

Remember, the path to chronic disease prevention and management is not a one-size-fits-all endeavor. Each individual's needs, risk factors, and personal circumstances may vary, requiring a tailored and adaptable approach. By working closely with healthcare providers, engaging in proactive self-care, and tapping into community resources, older adults can develop a personalized strategy that empowers them to address their unique health concerns and maintain their overall well-being.

Throughout this journey, it's essential to remain patient, persistent, and open-minded. Chronic disease prevention and management can be a complex and ever-evolving process, with ups and downs along the way. By celebrating small victories, learning from setbacks, and continuously seeking new ways to improve their health, older adults can foster a sense of resilience and ownership over their chronic condition management.

Ultimately, the prevention and management of chronic diseases is not just about addressing physical health challenges – it's about empowering older adults to live their best lives, maintain their independence, and create a lasting legacy of health and well-being. By embracing this holistic approach, we can redefine the narrative of aging, inspire others, and demonstrate the transformative power of proactive, comprehensive healthcare.

So, let's embark on this journey together, drawing upon the knowledge, strategies, and community support outlined in this chapter. By working in partnership with our healthcare providers, leveraging the resources available to us, and making healthy lifestyle choices a consistent part of our daily routines, we can unlock a world of possibilities and create a future where chronic diseases no longer define the aging experience.

CHAPTER 8

Chapter 8: Preventive Healthcare and Screenings

As we navigate the journey of healthy aging, one of the most crucial aspects of maintaining our well-being is a proactive, comprehensive approach to preventive healthcare. By prioritizing regular check-ups, screenings, and immunizations, we can take control of our health, detect potential issues early, and implement effective interventions to ensure a vibrant, independent, and resilient future.

In this chapter, we will explore the essential elements of preventive healthcare for older adults, delving into the recommended screening guidelines, the importance of immunizations, and strategies for creating a personalized healthcare plan that addresses your unique needs and goals. By embracing this holistic, preventive approach, you can empower yourself to take charge of your health and unlock the full potential of the golden years.

The Importance of Preventive Healthcare

Preventive healthcare is a fundamental pillar of healthy aging, as it enables us to identify and address potential health concerns before they escalate into more serious, debilitating conditions. By engaging in regular check-ups, screenings, and preventive measures, older adults can:

Early Detection and Intervention

Preventive healthcare allows for the early detection of various health issues, from chronic diseases to cancer. By catching these conditions in their earliest stages, older adults can often access more effective, less invasive interventions, leading to better outcomes and a higher quality of life.

Reduced Risk of Complications and Hospitalization

Proactive preventive care can help older adults avoid or manage chronic health conditions, ultimately reducing the risk of complications, hospitalizations, and the need for intensive medical treatment. This, in turn, can lead to greater independence, lower healthcare costs, and a decreased burden on the healthcare system.

Maintenance of Physical and Cognitive Function

Regular check-ups and screenings can help identify and address issues that may impact physical and cognitive function, such as vision and hearing problems, joint or muscle deterioration, or cognitive decline. By addressing these concerns early, older adults can maintain their independence, mobility, and mental acuity for longer.

Enhanced Emotional Well-being

Preventive healthcare also plays a role in supporting emotional well-being. By addressing physical health concerns proactively, older adults can reduce the stress and anxiety associated with health issues, fostering a greater sense of control and resilience.

Cost-effective Healthcare

Investing in preventive healthcare can actually save money in the long run by reducing the need for costly, late-stage medical interventions. By maintaining good health and catching issues early, older adults can minimize healthcare expenses and ensure a more financially secure future.

Recommended Preventive Screenings and Check-ups

To ensure optimal health and well-being, older adults should work closely with their healthcare providers to establish a personalized preventive healthcare plan that incorporates the recommended screenings and check-ups for their age group. While the specific recommendations may vary based on individual risk factors and health status, there are some essential preventive measures that all older adults should consider.

Cardiovascular Health Screenings

Regular cardiovascular health assessments are crucial for identifying and managing conditions such as high blood pressure, high cholesterol, and heart disease. Recommended screenings include:

- Blood pressure checks
    - Cholesterol tests
    - Electrocardiogram (ECG) to assess heart function
    - Screening for peripheral artery disease

Cancer Screenings

Early detection of various types of cancer can significantly improve outcomes and reduce the risk of complications. Common cancer screenings for older adults include:

- Mammograms for breast cancer
    - Colorectal cancer screenings (e.g., colonoscopy, stool-based tests)
    - Prostate cancer screenings for men (e.g., prostate-specific antigen (PSA) test)
    - Skin cancer examinations

Bone Health Assessments

Maintaining strong, healthy bones is essential for reducing the risk of falls and fractures, which can have a significant impact on older adults' independence and quality of life. Recommended bone health screenings include:

- Bone density scans (DXA or DEXA scans) to detect osteoporosis
    - Assessments of calcium and vitamin D levels

Cognitive and Neurological Evaluations

Regular cognitive and neurological assessments can help identify any potential issues, such as mild cognitive impairment or early-stage dementia, and implement appropriate interventions to support brain health. Recommended evaluations include:

- Cognitive function tests
    - Neuropsychological assessments
    - Screening for Parkinson's disease or other neurological conditions

Vision and Hearing Screenings

Maintaining good vision and hearing is crucial for older adults to navigate their daily lives safely and independently. Recommended screenings include:

- Eye exams to detect vision problems, cataracts, or glaucoma
    - Hearing tests to identify any hearing loss or impairment

Immunizations and Vaccinations

Staying up-to-date with recommended immunizations and vaccinations is an essential aspect of preventive healthcare for older adults, as their immune systems may be more vulnerable to certain infectious diseases. Some key vaccinations to consider include:

- Influenza (flu) vaccine
    - Pneumococcal vaccines
    - Shingles vaccine
    - Tetanus, diphtheria, and pertussis (Tdap) vaccine

It's important to note that the specific recommended screenings and vaccinations may vary based on individual health status, risk factors, and guidelines from trusted healthcare organizations, such as the Centers for Disease Control and Prevention (CDC) and the U.S. Preventive Services Task Force.

Creating a Personalized Preventive Healthcare Plan

While the recommended preventive screenings and check-ups provide a solid foundation for maintaining good health, it's essential for older adults to work closely with their healthcare providers to develop a personalized preventive healthcare plan that addresses their unique needs and goals.

Assess Individual Risk Factors

When creating a personalized preventive healthcare plan, it's crucial to consider individual risk factors that may influence the recommended screening and intervention strategies. These risk factors may include:

- Family medical history
    - Existing health conditions
    - Lifestyle factors (e.g., diet, physical activity, smoking status)
    - Environmental exposures
    - Socioeconomic status and access to healthcare

By thoroughly assessing these risk factors, healthcare providers can tailor the preventive healthcare plan to address any areas of heightened concern and ensure the most effective interventions are in place.

Establish Preventive Healthcare Goals

In collaboration with their healthcare providers, older adults should establish clear, measurable goals for their preventive healthcare plan. These goals may include:

- Maintaining or improving specific health metrics (e.g., blood pressure, cholesterol levels)
    - Reducing the risk of developing certain chronic conditions
    - Preserving physical and cognitive function
    - Enhancing emotional well-being and quality of life

By setting these personalized goals, older adults can stay motivated, track their progress, and make any necessary adjustments to their preventive healthcare strategies over time.

Develop a Comprehensive Care Plan

Based on the individual risk assessment and preventive healthcare goals, the healthcare provider and older adult can work together to develop a comprehensive care plan that includes:

- Recommended screenings and check-ups, along with the frequency and timing of each
    - Any necessary diagnostic tests or imaging procedures
    - Strategies for managing identified health risks or existing conditions
    - Referrals to specialists or other healthcare providers, as needed
    - Lifestyle modifications, such as dietary changes or increased physical activity
    - Immunization and vaccination schedule

This comprehensive care plan should be reviewed and updated regularly, as older adults' health needs and risk factors may change over time.

Ensure Ongoing Communication and Coordination

Effective preventive healthcare requires ongoing communication and co-ordination between the older adult and their healthcare team. This may involve:

- Regular check-ins with the primary care provider to discuss any changes or concerns
    - Timely scheduling of recommended screenings and check-ups
    - Sharing of test results and healthcare information with all members of the care team
    - Proactive outreach from healthcare providers to remind older adults of upcoming appointments or due dates for screenings

By maintaining open lines of communication and ensuring seamless coordination of care, older adults can feel empowered to take an active role in their preventive healthcare and stay on track with their personalized care plan.

Overcoming Barriers to Preventive Healthcare

While the benefits of preventive healthcare for older adults are well-established, there may be various barriers and challenges that can hinder their ability to access and engage with these essential services. Understanding and addressing these barriers is crucial for ensuring that all older adults can take advantage of the opportunities for early detection, intervention, and maintenance of good health.

Limited Access to Healthcare

One of the primary barriers to preventive healthcare for older adults, particularly those with lower incomes or living in underserved communities, is limited access to healthcare services. This may include:

- Lack of transportation or mobility issues that make it difficult to attend appointments
    - Financial constraints that make it challenging to afford healthcare costs, including copays and deductibles
    - Shortages of healthcare providers, especially in certain geographical areas, leading to long wait times or limited availability

To overcome these access barriers, older adults can explore community resources, such as transportation assistance programs, sliding-scale or free clinics, and telehealth services that can bring healthcare directly to their homes.

Fears and Misconceptions

Some older adults may be hesitant to engage in preventive healthcare due to fears, misconceptions, or lack of understanding about the importance of these services. These concerns may include:

- Fear of receiving a serious diagnosis or prognosis
    - Belief that preventive screenings are unnecessary or not worth the time and effort
    - Misconceptions about the costs or accessibility of preventive healthcare services

To address these fears and misconceptions, healthcare providers can take a proactive role in educating older adults about the benefits of preventive care, addressing their concerns, and emphasizing the importance of early detection and intervention.

Lack of Awareness or Motivation

In some cases, older adults may simply be unaware of the recommended preventive healthcare guidelines or lack the motivation to prioritize these services amid the demands of daily life. This can be particularly challenging for older adults who may have limited access to information or who are dealing with cognitive or physical impairments.

To raise awareness and boost motivation, healthcare providers can leverage various strategies, such as:

- Providing clear, easy-to-understand educational materials about preventive healthcare
    - Implementing patient-centered appointment reminders and scheduling systems
    - Collaborating with community organizations to promote preventive healthcare services
    - Encouraging older adults to involve their families or caregivers in their healthcare decisions and planning

By addressing these barriers and empowering older adults to take a proactive role in their preventive healthcare, we can ensure that all individuals have the opportunity to maintain their health, independence, and quality of life throughout the golden years.

Embracing a Holistic Approach to Preventive Healthcare

Preventive healthcare is a fundamental pillar of healthy aging, providing older adults with the tools and strategies to detect, manage, and even prevent a wide range of health issues. By embracing a comprehensive, holistic approach to preventive care, older adults can optimize their physical, cognitive, and emotional well-being, ultimately enhancing their independence, resilience, and quality of life.

Remember, preventive healthcare is not a one-time event, but rather an ongoing process that requires commitment, collaboration, and a willingness to adapt to changing needs and circumstances. By working closely with their healthcare providers, staying up-to-date with recommended screenings and vaccinations, and incorporating preventive strategies into their daily lives, older adults can create a personalized plan that addresses their unique health concerns and supports their long-term well-being.

Moreover, preventive healthcare is not just about individual benefits – it can also have a positive impact on the broader healthcare system and community. By proactively managing their health, older adults can reduce the burden on healthcare resources, lower healthcare costs, and inspire others to take a more active role in their own preventive care.

As you embark on this journey of preventive healthcare, be patient, persistent, and open to trying new approaches. Celebrate your successes, learn from any setbacks, and remain flexible in your approach, as your healthcare needs may evolve over time. Remember that you are not alone in this process – reach out to your healthcare providers, community resources, and support networks to build a strong foundation for your preventive care.

Ultimately, embracing preventive healthcare is an investment in your future, a commitment to maintaining your independence, and a testament to your dedication to living a vibrant, fulfilled life. By taking control of your health and prioritizing these essential preventive measures, you can unlock a world of possibilities and create a lasting legacy of well-being that inspires and empowers those around you.

So, let's dive in, explore the preventive healthcare strategies and resources that resonate most with you, and embark on a journey of proactive, comprehensive healthcare. Together, we can redefine the aging experience and demonstrate the transformative power of preventive care.

CHAPTER 9

hapter 9: Supplements and Holistic Approaches

As we navigate the journey of healthy aging, it's important to recognize that a comprehensive approach to well-being often involves exploring a range of complementary strategies and therapies, in addition to conventional medical care. While maintaining a balanced, nutrient-dense diet and adhering to prescribed treatments are essential, the strategic use of nutritional supplements and the integration of holistic practices can provide an additional layer of support for older adults seeking to optimize their physical, cognitive, and emotional health.

In this chapter, we will delve into the world of supplements and holistic approaches, examining the potential benefits, risks, and considerations for older adults. We will explore evidence-based recommendations, dispel common myths, and provide guidance on how to incorporate these complementary strategies into a well-rounded, personalized plan for healthy aging.

The Role of Nutritional Supplements

Nutritional supplements can play a valuable role in supporting the health and well-being of older adults, particularly in situations where dietary intake alone may not be sufficient to meet their unique nutrient needs. However, it's essential to approach the use of supplements with caution, as they can interact with medications or have other potential side effects, especially for older individuals.

Understanding Nutrient Needs in Older Adults

As we age, our bodies' ability to absorb and utilize certain nutrients can diminish, making it more challenging to meet our daily requirements through diet alone. Some of the key nutrients that older adults may struggle to obtain in sufficient quantities include:

- Vitamin B12: Reduced stomach acid production can impair the absorption of this essential vitamin, which is crucial for red blood cell formation and neurological function.
  - Vitamin D: Decreased sun exposure and the skin's capacity to synthesize vitamin D can lead to deficiencies, which are linked to bone health and immune function.
  - Calcium: Decreased absorption and increased excretion of calcium can contribute to the development of osteoporosis, a common condition in older adults.
  - Omega-3 fatty acids: Older adults may have a higher risk of cardiovascular disease and cognitive decline, making adequate intake of these beneficial fats important.

In addition to these specific nutrients, older adults may also face challenges in meeting their overall protein, fiber, and hydration needs, further highlighting the potential role of targeted supplementation.

Evidence-based Supplement Recommendations

While the use of supplements should always be discussed with a healthcare provider, there are certain evidence-based supplements that may benefit older adults when used judiciously and under medical supervision. Some of the more well-studied and potentially beneficial supplements include:

- Multivitamin: A comprehensive multivitamin can help fill any nutrient gaps in the diet and provide a broad range of essential vitamins and minerals.
- Vitamin B12: Older adults may benefit from B12 supplements, especially if they have been diagnosed with a deficiency or have conditions that impair absorption.
- Vitamin D: Vitamin D supplements can help maintain bone health and support immune function, particularly for those with limited sun exposure.
- Calcium: Calcium supplements, often combined with vitamin D, can help prevent or manage osteoporosis.
- Omega-3 fatty acids: Fish oil or algae-based supplements can provide a concentrated source of heart-healthy omega-3s.
- Probiotics: These beneficial gut bacteria can support digestive health and immune function in older adults.

It's important to note that the appropriate type, dosage, and timing of supplements can vary depending on an individual's health status, medication use, and overall dietary intake. Working closely with a healthcare provider is crucial to ensure the safe and effective use of any supplementation.

Addressing Supplement Risks and Interactions

While supplements can provide valuable support for older adults, it's essential to be aware of the potential risks and interactions associated with their use. Some key considerations include:

- Interactions with medications: Certain supplements, such as St. John's wort or ginkgo biloba, can interact with prescription drugs, potentially altering their effectiveness or causing adverse effects.
- Potential side effects: Even seemingly benign supplements can cause unwanted side effects, particularly when taken in excess or without proper guidance.
- Quality and safety concerns: The supplement industry is largely unregulated, so it's important to source products from reputable manufacturers and

be wary of false claims or adulterated products.

To mitigate these risks, older adults should always consult with their healthcare providers before starting any new supplement regimen, provide a comprehensive list of their current medications and supplements, and carefully follow the recommended dosages and usage instructions.

Integrating Holistic Approaches

In addition to the strategic use of nutritional supplements, older adults may also benefit from the integration of various holistic and complementary therapies into their overall wellness plan. These holistic approaches can provide a multifaceted support system for physical, cognitive, and emotional well-being, often in a way that complements conventional medical care.

Mind-body Practices

Techniques that focus on the connection between the mind and body can be particularly beneficial for older adults, as they can help manage stress, improve emotional regulation, and enhance overall well-being. Some popular mind-body practices include:

- Meditation and mindfulness: These practices can help reduce stress, improve cognitive function, and promote a sense of inner calm.
  - Yoga and Tai Chi: These gentle, low-impact forms of exercise incorporate breathing, movement, and mental focus, which can improve balance, flexibility, and relaxation.
  - Guided imagery and visualization: These techniques can help manage pain, reduce anxiety, and promote healing.

By incorporating these mind-body practices into their daily routines, older adults can cultivate a greater sense of emotional resilience, physical well-being, and overall quality of life.

Herbal and Botanical Remedies

Certain herbal and botanical preparations have been used for centuries to support various aspects of health and well-being. While the scientific evidence for the efficacy of many herbal remedies is still evolving, some show potential benefits for older adults, such as:

- Ginkgo biloba: This herb is often used to support cognitive function and may help improve memory and concentration.
   - Turmeric: The active compound in turmeric, curcumin, has been studied for its anti-inflammatory and neuroprotective properties, which may benefit older adults.
   - Valerian: This herb is sometimes used to support sleep quality and manage anxiety or insomnia.

It's important to note that, like supplements, herbal and botanical remedies can interact with medications and have potential side effects, particularly for older adults. Therefore, it's crucial to consult with a healthcare provider before incorporating these therapies into one's wellness plan.

Energy Therapies

Energy therapies, such as acupuncture, reiki, and therapeutic touch, focus on the manipulation or balancing of the body's energy fields to promote healing and well-being. While the scientific mechanisms behind these practices are still being explored, some studies have suggested potential benefits for older adults, including:

- Pain management: Acupuncture and related therapies may help alleviate chronic pain conditions, such as osteoarthritis or neuropathic pain.
   - Improved sleep and relaxation: Energy therapies may help reduce stress and promote better sleep quality.
   - Enhanced emotional well-being: These practices may help manage

anxiety, depression, and other emotional health concerns.

As with other holistic approaches, it's essential for older adults to work with qualified practitioners and disclose any existing health conditions or medication use to ensure the safe and effective integration of these therapies.

Nutrition and Dietary Approaches

In addition to the strategic use of supplements, older adults may also benefit from exploring various dietary approaches and nutritional therapies that can support their overall health and well-being. These may include:

- Therapeutic diets: Specific dietary patterns, such as the Mediterranean diet or the DASH diet, have been associated with a lower risk of chronic diseases and cognitive decline.
  - Functional foods and nutraceuticals: Certain food-based compounds, such as probiotics, antioxidants, and anti-inflammatory agents, may provide targeted health benefits when incorporated into the diet.
  - Personalized nutrition: Advances in nutrigenomics and personalized medicine can help identify individualized dietary needs and optimize nutrient intake.

By working with healthcare providers or registered dietitians who specialize in geriatric nutrition, older adults can develop a personalized dietary plan that nourishes their bodies, supports their health goals, and complements any other medical or holistic therapies they may be pursuing.

Balancing Conventional and Holistic Approaches

As we navigate the world of supplements and holistic therapies, it's essential to recognize that they should not be viewed as a replacement for conventional medical care, but rather as a complement to it. The most effective approach to healthy aging often involves a carefully balanced integration of both traditional and complementary strategies, with the guidance of healthcare professionals.

Communicating with Healthcare Providers

When incorporating supplements or holistic therapies into their wellness plan, older adults should always be transparent and communicative with their healthcare providers. This includes:

- Providing a comprehensive list of all supplements, herbs, and other holistic therapies they are using or considering
    - Discussing the potential benefits, risks, and interactions associated with these complementary approaches
    - Seeking guidance on the appropriate timing, dosage, and integration of supplements and holistic therapies with any existing medical treatments

By working closely with their healthcare team, older adults can ensure that their use of supplements and holistic approaches is safe, effective, and aligned with their overall health goals.

Evaluating Evidence and Reputable Sources

With the abundance of information (and misinformation) available regarding supplements and holistic therapies, it's crucial for older adults to carefully evaluate the evidence and sources behind any claims or recommendations. When exploring these complementary approaches, they should:

- Refer to trusted, evidence-based resources, such as those provided by government health agencies, academic institutions, or reputable healthcare organizations.
    - Be wary of unsubstantiated claims, particularly those made by commercial entities with a vested interest in selling specific products or services.
    - Consult with healthcare providers who are knowledgeable about integra-

tive and holistic approaches, as they can provide informed guidance on the appropriate use of these therapies.

By conducting thorough research and relying on credible sources, older adults can make informed decisions about the supplements and holistic approaches that are most likely to benefit their health and well-being.

Adopting a Collaborative, Adaptive Approach

Ultimately, the most effective approach to incorporating supplements and holistic therapies into a healthy aging plan involves a collaborative, adaptive mindset. Older adults should work closely with their healthcare providers to:

- Develop a personalized, integrated wellness plan that balances conventional and complementary strategies
  - Monitor the effects of any supplements or holistic therapies, making adjustments as needed based on their individual responses and evolving health needs
  - Stay open to exploring new evidence-based approaches and be willing to try different combinations of therapies to find what works best for them

By embracing this collaborative, adaptive approach, older adults can create a comprehensive, personalized wellness strategy that harnesses the benefits of both conventional and complementary therapies, empowering them to optimize their physical, cognitive, and emotional well-being throughout the golden years.

Embracing the Power of Integrative Wellness

As we have explored in this chapter, the strategic use of supplements and the integration of holistic approaches can play a valuable role in supporting the health and well-being of older adults. By recognizing the limitations of a one-size-fits-all approach to healthcare and embracing the potential benefits of these complementary strategies, we can empower older adults to take a more active, personalized role in their own wellness journey.

Remember, the path to integrative wellness is not a simple or linear one. It requires a willingness to experiment, adapt, and collaborate with healthcare providers to find the right balance of conventional and complementary therapies. Along the way, there may be successes and setbacks, but by remaining open-minded, persistent, and attentive to your body's unique needs, you can navigate this journey with confidence and resilience.

Ultimately, the integration of supplements and holistic approaches into a healthy aging plan is not about abandoning traditional medical care, but rather about creating a comprehensive, multifaceted approach to well-being. By harnessing the potential benefits of these complementary strategies, while maintaining open communication and collaboration with healthcare providers, older adults can unlock a world of possibilities and enhance their overall quality of life.

As you embark on this journey of integrative wellness, remember that you are not alone. Reach out to your healthcare team, support networks, and the larger community of older adults who are also exploring the power of complementary therapies. Together, we can create a culture of healthy aging that celebrates the diverse array of tools and approaches available for optimizing physical, cognitive, and emotional well-being.

So, let us dive in, explore the supplements and holistic practices that resonate most with you, and embrace the transformative potential of integrative wellness. The future is bright, and it starts with a balanced, personalized approach to your health and well-being.

CHAPTER 10

Chapter 10: Age-Friendly Environments and Accessibility

As we navigate the journey of healthy aging, the environments in which we live, work, and play play a crucial role in supporting our independence, mobility, and overall quality of life. From our homes to our communities, the accessibility and adaptability of our surroundings can have a profound impact on our ability to safely and comfortably engage in daily activities, pursue our passions, and maintain a sense of autonomy.

In this chapter, we will explore the concept of age-friendly environments and delve into the strategies and resources available to help older adults create living spaces, public spaces, and transportation systems that cater to their unique needs and preferences. By understanding the importance of accessibility and adaptability, we can empower ourselves to design a lifestyle that enables us to thrive in the golden years and beyond.

The Importance of Age-Friendly Environments

As we grow older, our physical, sensory, and cognitive needs can evolve, requiring us to adapt our living environments and the public spaces we navigate. Age-friendly environments are designed to prioritize the accessibility, safety, and overall well-being of older adults, helping them to maintain their independence, participate in their communities, and enjoy a higher quality of life.

Promoting Independence and Mobility

One of the primary benefits of age-friendly environments is their ability to support the independence and mobility of older adults. By incorporating features such as barrier-free access, ergonomic design, and assistive technologies, these environments can enable older adults to safely navigate their surroundings, perform daily tasks, and engage in the activities they enjoy without relying on constant assistance or the risk of falls or injuries.

This enhanced independence and mobility, in turn, can have a positive impact on an older adult's emotional well-being, self-confidence, and sense of control over their own lives, ultimately contributing to their overall health and quality of life.

Reducing the Risk of Accidents and Injuries

As we age, our risk of falls, accidents, and other safety-related incidents can increase due to factors such as reduced mobility, impaired vision or hearing, and cognitive changes. Age-friendly environments, however, are designed with these considerations in mind, incorporating features that help to mitigate these risks and promote a safer living and community experience.

This can include elements like non-slip flooring, adequate lighting, handrails, and clear visual cues – all of which can significantly reduce the likelihood of accidents and injuries among older adults. By creating these safer environments, we can help older adults maintain their physical well-being, avoid costly and debilitating healthcare interventions, and continue to engage in their daily activities with confidence and peace of mind.

Supporting Aging in Place and Community Involvement

Another key benefit of age-friendly environments is their ability to support older adults' desire to age in place – that is, to remain living independently in their own homes and communities for as long as possible. By ensuring that the places we live, work, and play are accessible and adaptable to our changing needs, we can empower older adults to continue participating in their local communities, accessing essential services, and maintaining their social connections.

This, in turn, can foster a greater sense of belonging, purpose, and overall well-being, as older adults are able to remain actively engaged in the neighborhoods and social networks that are familiar and meaningful to them. Furthermore, age-friendly communities can help to reduce the need for institutionalized care, such as nursing homes or assisted living facilities, allowing older adults to maintain their autonomy and independence for longer.

Enhancing Inclusivity and Community Cohesion

Finally, the creation of age-friendly environments can have a positive impact on the broader community, promoting inclusivity and fostering a greater sense of cohesion among individuals of all ages. By designing public spaces, transportation systems, and community services that cater to the needs of older adults, we can ensure that everyone, regardless of their age or ability level, can participate in and contribute to the vibrancy of their local communities.

This inclusive approach not only benefits older adults but also creates opportunities for intergenerational connections, understanding, and mutual support. As people of all ages are able to comfortably and safely navigate their shared spaces, they can engage in meaningful interactions, share experiences, and develop a deeper appreciation for the diverse needs and perspectives within their communities.

Adapting Your Home for Healthy Aging

One of the most critical aspects of age-friendly environments is the home, where older adults spend a significant portion of their time and where the need for accessibility and adaptability is paramount. By incorporating age-friendly design principles and modifications into our living spaces, we can create a sanctuary that supports our physical, cognitive, and emotional well-being as we grow older.

Evaluating and Addressing Accessibility Needs

The first step in adapting your home for healthy aging is to conduct a thorough assessment of your current living environment, identifying any potential accessibility challenges or safety hazards. This can involve considering factors such as:

- Ease of entry and movement within the home (e.g., doorways, hallways, stairs)
    - Bathroom safety and functionality (e.g., tub/shower, toilets, sinks)
    - Kitchen ergonomics and task-oriented design
    - Lighting, both natural and artificial, to enhance visibility
    - Flooring materials and traction to prevent falls
    - Smart home technologies and assistive devices

By addressing these accessibility needs through home modifications, older adults can create a living space that enables them to move around safely, maintain their independence, and continue engaging in the activities they enjoy.

Incorporating Universal Design Principles

In addition to addressing specific accessibility requirements, the incorporation of universal design principles can further enhance the adaptability and inclusivity of a home environment. Universal design is an approach that aims to create spaces that are usable by all people, to the greatest extent possible, without the need for adaptation or specialized design.

Some key universal design features that can benefit older adults include:

- Wider doorways and hallways to accommodate mobility aids
    - Single-level living with no steps or split levels
    - Adjustable-height countertops and cabinets
    - Lever-style door handles and faucets
    - Flexible seating options, such as height-adjustable chairs
    - Integrated smart home technologies for remote control and monitoring

By embracing these universal design principles, older adults can future-proof their homes, ensuring that their living spaces remain accessible and adaptable as their needs evolve over time.

Leveraging Community Resources and Assistance

For older adults who may require additional support or expertise in adapting their homes, a range of community resources and assistance programs are often available. These can include:

- Local government or non-profit organizations that offer home modification grants or subsidies
    - Occupational therapists or aging-in-place specialists who can provide personalized assessments and recommendations
    - Volunteer programs or handyman services that assist with the physical installation of accessibility features
    - Educational workshops or online resources that guide older adults through the home modification process

By tapping into these community-based resources, older adults can access the necessary information, funding, and practical support to create a home environment that truly meets their needs and empowers them to age in place with confidence.

Navigating Public Spaces and Transportation

While the home is a crucial component of an age-friendly environment, older adults also need to be able to safely and comfortably navigate the public spaces and transportation systems within their communities. By advocating for and utilizing age-friendly features in these broader settings, older adults can maintain their independence, access essential services, and continue participating in the social and civic life of their neighborhoods.

Ensuring Accessibility in Public Spaces

When it comes to public spaces, such as parks, libraries, shopping centers, or government buildings, older adults should look for the following accessibility features:

- Clearly marked and level pathways, with minimal steps or curbs
    - Ample seating options, including benches with backrests and armrests
    - Accessible restrooms equipped with grab bars and wide stall doors
    - Signage and wayfinding cues that are easy to read and understand
    - Tactile paving, audio cues, and other sensory aids for individuals with visual or hearing impairments

By advocating for the inclusion of these age-friendly design elements in public spaces, older adults can feel confident and safe as they navigate their local communities, engage in recreational activities, and access the services and amenities they require.

Utilizing Age-friendly Transportation Options

Maintaining the ability to travel and access transportation is crucial for older adults to remain independent, connected, and engaged with their communities. Age-friendly transportation options can include:

- Public transit systems with accessible features, such as low-floor buses, ramps, and priority seating
    - Paratransit or demand-responsive services that provide door-to-door transportation for older adults and individuals with disabilities
    - Ridesharing or volunteer driver programs that offer personalized transportation assistance
    - Community-based shuttle services or mobility programs tailored to the needs of older adults

In addition to these transportation options, older adults should also consider the accessibility of the built environment surrounding transportation hubs, such as well-lit and level walkways, appropriate signage, and the availability of benches or shelters.

By utilizing a combination of these age-friendly transportation resources, older adults can maintain their independence, access essential services and social activities, and continue participating in the life of their communities.

Advocating for Age-friendly Community Design

While individual home and transportation adaptations are crucial, the development of truly age-friendly communities also requires a broader, collaborative approach that involves advocacy, policy-making, and community engagement. Older adults can play a vital role in this process by:

- Participating in local government planning initiatives or community task forces focused on age-friendly design
    - Providing input and feedback to policymakers, urban planners, and community leaders on the unique needs and priorities of older adults
    - Collaborating with local organizations, businesses, and service providers to promote the integration of age-friendly features and practices

- Raising awareness and educating the broader community about the importance of accessible, adaptable, and inclusive public spaces

By actively engaging in these community-level initiatives, older adults can help to shape the built environment and ensure that their local neighborhoods are designed to support healthy aging, increase social participation, and enhance the quality of life for people of all ages.

Accessing Community Resources and Support Services

In addition to the physical design and accessibility of our living environments, older adults can also benefit from a robust network of community resources and support services that cater to their unique needs and preferences. By tapping into these local and regional offerings, older adults can maintain their independence, access essential services, and engage in fulfilling activities.

Identifying and Utilizing Community Resources

Some examples of community resources and support services that can benefit older adults include:

- Senior centers or community centers that provide social activities, educational programs, and recreational opportunities
  - Meal delivery services or community-based nutrition programs to support healthy eating
  - Transportation assistance, such as ride-sharing programs or volunteer driver networks
  - In-home care services, including personal care, housekeeping, or nursing support
  - Local libraries, museums, or cultural institutions that offer specialized programming for older adults

By researching and taking advantage of these community-based resources, older adults can enhance their quality of life, maintain their independence, and feel more connected to their local communities.

Navigating Government Benefits and Entitlements

Older adults may also be eligible for a range of government benefits and entitlements that can help support their health, financial security, and overall well-being. These can include:

- Medicare and Medicaid coverage for healthcare services
    - Social Security retirement or disability benefits
    - Supplemental Security Income (SSI) for individuals with limited income and resources
    - Veteran's benefits for older adults who have served in the military
    - Property tax or utility bill assistance programs for low-income older adults

Navigating the complexities of these government programs can be challenging, which is why older adults should seek the guidance of local social service organizations, financial advisors, or community outreach professionals who can help them identify and access the benefits they are entitled to.

Engaging with Community-Based Organizations and Advocacy Groups

In addition to government-provided resources, older adults can also benefit from connecting with community-based organizations and advocacy groups that champion the needs and interests of the aging population. These can include:

- Local chapters of national aging advocacy organizations, such as AARP or the Alzheimer's Association
    - Community-based non-profit organizations that provide support services, educational programs, or social activities for older adults

- Neighborhood or resident associations that advocate for age-friendly community design and policies

By engaging with these groups, older adults can not only access valuable resources and support but also have a voice in shaping the policies, services, and environments that impact their daily lives.

Embracing the Power of Age-Friendly Environments and Accessibility

As we have explored in this chapter, the creation of age-friendly environments and the promotion of accessibility are crucial components of healthy aging. By adapting our living spaces, navigating public spaces and transportation, and tapping into community resources, we can empower ourselves to maintain our independence, participate in our communities, and enjoy a higher quality of life throughout the golden years.

Remember, the pursuit of age-friendly environments is not a solitary endeavor – it requires collaboration, advocacy, and a collective commitment to creating inclusive, accessible, and supportive communities for people of all ages and abilities. By engaging with local government, community organizations, and our fellow citizens, we can shape the built environment and the services that cater to the unique needs and preferences of older adults.

Moreover, the benefits of age-friendly environments extend beyond the individual – they have the power to enhance the overall cohesion and vibrancy of our communities. By designing spaces and services that are inclusive and accessible, we can foster greater intergenerational understanding, reduce social isolation, and promote the active participation of older adults in the civic and social life of their neighborhoods.

As you navigate this journey of healthy aging, remember to be patient, persistent, and open to exploring new resources and strategies. Celebrate your successes, learn from any setbacks, and remain flexible in your approach, as your needs and preferences may change over time. Reach out to your support networks, community organizations, and fellow older adults who are also committed to creating age-friendly environments and promoting accessibility.

Ultimately, the pursuit of age-friendly environments is not just about adapting our physical surroundings – it's about empowering ourselves to live with greater independence, dignity, and purpose. By embracing this holistic approach to healthy aging, we can unlock a world of possibilities, inspire others, and leave a lasting legacy that positively impacts the lives of older adults for generations to come.

So, let's dive in, explore the resources and strategies that resonate most with you, and embark on a journey of creating age-friendly environments and accessible communities that support our well-being and empower us to thrive in the golden years and beyond.

CHAPTER 11

C hapter 11: Financial Planning and Retirement

As we navigate the journey of healthy aging, it's essential to recognize that our financial well-being plays a crucial role in our overall quality of life and our ability to thrive in the golden years. From ensuring a secure retirement income to managing healthcare costs, our financial decisions and planning can have a profound impact on our physical, emotional, and social well-being.

In this chapter, we will explore the key aspects of financial planning and retirement for older adults, providing you with the knowledge and strategies to create a solid financial foundation that supports your healthy aging goals. By taking a proactive, comprehensive approach to your financial future, you can empower yourself to enjoy a fulfilling, independent, and financially secure retirement.

Preparing for a Secure Financial Future

Achieving a financially secure retirement is a fundamental aspect of healthy aging, as it allows older adults to maintain their independence, address their healthcare needs, and pursue the activities and lifestyle they desire. Effective financial planning involves a multi-faceted approach that addresses various considerations, from saving and investing to navigating government benefits and healthcare costs.

Building a Robust Retirement Savings Plan

The foundation of a secure financial future is a well-designed retirement savings plan. This may include a combination of the following:

- Employer-sponsored retirement accounts (e.g., 401(k), 403(b), or pension plans)
    - Individual retirement accounts (IRAs), such as traditional or Roth IRAs
    - Taxable investment accounts, such as brokerage or mutual fund accounts

By contributing consistently to these retirement savings vehicles, older adults can take advantage of tax-deferred or tax-free growth, employer matching contributions, and the power of compound interest to build a robust nest egg.

It's important to note that the specific retirement savings strategies may vary based on individual circumstances, such as income, tax status, and access to employer-sponsored plans. Consulting with a qualified financial advisor can help older adults develop a personalized retirement savings plan that aligns with their goals and risk tolerance.

Maximizing Government Benefits and Entitlements

In addition to personal retirement savings, older adults should also explore and maximize the various government benefits and entitlements available to them, such as:

- Social Security: Understanding the optimal time to claim Social Security benefits and strategies to maximize these payments can have a significant impact on retirement income.
    - Medicare: Navigating the complexities of Medicare coverage and supplemental insurance can help older adults manage healthcare costs.
    - Veteran's benefits: Older adults who have served in the military may be

eligible for a range of benefits, including healthcare, disability, and retirement income.

- Supplemental Security Income (SSI) and Medicaid: These programs can provide financial assistance and healthcare coverage for older adults with limited income and assets.

By thoroughly understanding and strategically utilizing these government benefits, older adults can enhance their financial security and quality of life in retirement.

Managing Healthcare Costs and Long-Term Care

One of the most significant financial considerations for older adults is the cost of healthcare and long-term care. As we age, the likelihood of developing chronic health conditions or requiring long-term care services increases, which can place a substantial burden on personal finances.

To address these healthcare-related costs, older adults should consider the following strategies:

- Comprehensive health insurance coverage: Ensuring adequate medical insurance, including Medicare, supplemental plans, and prescription drug coverage, can help mitigate out-of-pocket expenses.
- Long-term care insurance: Purchasing long-term care insurance can provide financial protection against the high costs of in-home care, assisted living, or nursing home services.
- Healthcare savings accounts: Utilizing tax-advantaged healthcare savings accounts, such as Health Savings Accounts (HSAs) or Flexible Spending Accounts (FSAs), can help cover medical expenses.
- Budgeting and cost management: Carefully managing healthcare-related expenses, including prescription medications and out-of-pocket costs, can help older adults maintain financial stability.

By proactively addressing healthcare costs and long-term care needs, older adults can ensure that their financial resources are optimized to support their health and well-being throughout retirement.

Navigating the Retirement Transition

Retirement is a significant life transition that can bring with it a range of emotional, social, and financial adjustments. Effective retirement planning not only involves the financial aspects but also encompasses the psychological and lifestyle changes that often accompany this next chapter of life.

Retirement Income Planning

One of the key aspects of retirement planning is ensuring a reliable and sustainable income stream. This may involve a combination of the following strategies:

- Calculating retirement income needs: Estimating essential expenses, such as housing, food, and healthcare, as well as discretionary spending, can help older adults determine the required retirement income.
  - Diversifying income sources: Relying on a mix of income sources, such as Social Security, pension plans, retirement account withdrawals, and investment returns, can provide more stability and flexibility.
  - Optimizing Social Security and pension benefits: Developing a strategic plan for when to claim Social Security and how to maximize pension benefits can significantly impact retirement income.
  - Managing retirement account withdrawals: Carefully planning for the withdrawal of funds from retirement accounts, such as 401(k)s and IRAs, can help older adults minimize taxes and ensure their savings last throughout retirement.

By carefully planning and managing their retirement income, older adults can create a more secure and sustainable financial foundation for their golden years.

Lifestyle and Emotional Adjustments

In addition to the financial aspects of retirement, older adults must also navigate the emotional and lifestyle changes that come with this transition. Some key considerations include:

- Maintaining a sense of purpose and fulfillment: Retirement can present an opportunity to explore new hobbies, volunteer, or pursue encore careers, which can help older adults find meaning and purpose in this next chapter of life.
  - Adapting to changes in social networks and relationships: Retirement can impact an individual's social connections, as they may no longer have the same daily interactions with colleagues or regular routines. Older adults should proactively cultivate new social connections and maintain existing relationships.
  - Managing the psychological and emotional aspects of retirement: The transition to retirement can trigger a range of emotions, from excitement and relief to anxiety and boredom. Older adults should be prepared to address these emotional adjustments and seek support if needed.

By addressing the emotional and lifestyle aspects of retirement, older adults can ensure a smoother transition and a more fulfilling, well-rounded retirement experience.

Considerations for Encore Careers and Part-time Work

For some older adults, retirement may not mean a complete withdrawal from the workforce. Many choose to pursue encore careers or part-time work, either out of financial necessity or a desire to remain engaged and active. When considering these options, older adults should carefully evaluate the following:

- Potential impact on retirement income and benefits: Earning income from employment may affect Social Security, pension, or other retirement benefits, so it's essential to understand the financial implications.
 - Availability of employer-sponsored health insurance: For those not yet eligible for Medicare, maintaining health insurance coverage through an employer-sponsored plan can be a crucial consideration.
 - Work-life balance and personal fulfillment: Older adults should strike a balance between their financial needs, desired lifestyle, and the level of engagement they seek from any post-retirement work.

By thoughtfully evaluating the pros and cons of encore careers or part-time work, older adults can make informed decisions that align with their overall retirement goals and well-being.

Strategies for Retirement Financial Security

Achieving a financially secure retirement requires a multifaceted approach that addresses various aspects of financial planning, investment management, and risk mitigation. By incorporating the following strategies, older adults can create a solid foundation for their golden years.

Diversifying Investment Portfolios

Diversification is a fundamental principle of sound investment management, as it helps to mitigate risk and ensure a more stable, resilient portfolio. For older adults, a well-diversified investment portfolio may include a mix of the following:

- Stocks (including domestic and international equities)
 - Bonds (government, corporate, and municipal bonds)
 - Real estate (such as investment properties or real estate investment trusts)
 - Alternative investments (e.g., commodities, precious metals, hedge funds)

By allocating assets across various sectors and asset classes, older adults can reduce their exposure to market volatility and safeguard their retirement savings.

Preserving Capital and Generating Income

In retirement, the focus often shifts from capital appreciation to preserving wealth and generating a reliable income stream. Strategies to achieve this include:

- Allocating a portion of the portfolio to fixed-income investments, such as bonds or annuities, to provide a steady stream of income.
    - Utilizing withdrawal strategies, such as the 4% rule or the "bucket" approach, to manage the systematic withdrawal of retirement savings in a tax-efficient manner.
    - Considering the use of reverse mortgages or home equity lines of credit to access the equity in one's home, if appropriate.

By carefully balancing the need for growth and income, older adults can create a retirement income plan that supports their long-term financial security.

Minimizing Taxes and Managing Distributions

Effective tax planning is a crucial component of retirement financial security, as it can help older adults maximize their retirement income and minimize their tax burden. Strategies to consider include:

- Optimizing the timing and distribution of retirement account withdrawals (e.g., 401(k)s, IRAs) to manage income tax liability.
    - Utilizing tax-advantaged investment vehicles, such as Roth IRAs or tax-efficient mutual funds, to generate tax-free or tax-deferred growth.
    - Carefully managing the taxation of Social Security benefits and other income sources to ensure efficient tax planning.

- Exploring estate planning strategies, such as trusts or charitable giving, to minimize the impact of estate and gift taxes.

By proactively addressing tax-related considerations, older adults can preserve a greater portion of their retirement savings and enhance their long-term financial security.

Protecting Against Financial Risks

Retirement financial planning should also include strategies to mitigate various risks that can threaten an individual's financial well-being, such as:

- Longevity risk: The risk of outliving one's retirement savings, which can be addressed through prudent withdrawal strategies and longevity insurance (e.g., annuities).
  - Health and long-term care risks: Comprehensive health insurance coverage, including Medicare and long-term care insurance, can help protect against the high costs of healthcare and long-term care services.
  - Market risks: Diversification, risk management techniques, and the use of guaranteed income products can help mitigate the impact of market volatility on retirement savings.
  - Fraud and financial exploitation: Vigilance, financial literacy, and the involvement of trusted family members or advisors can help older adults protect against financial scams and exploitation.

By addressing these potential financial risks, older adults can create a more secure and resilient retirement plan that safeguards their hard-earned savings and ensures their long-term financial well-being.

Embracing a Holistic Approach to Retirement Planning

Effective retirement planning is not just about the financial aspects – it's about creating a comprehensive, holistic strategy that addresses the various facets of healthy aging, including physical, emotional, and social well-being. By integrating these elements into their retirement planning, older adults can ensure a fulfilling, independent, and financially secure future.

Aligning Financial Goals with Healthy Aging Priorities

When developing a retirement plan, it's essential for older adults to align their financial goals with their broader healthy aging priorities. This may involve:

- Budgeting for healthcare expenses and preventive care to maintain physical and cognitive health
    - Allocating resources to support social engagement, lifelong learning, and other activities that promote emotional well-being
    - Ensuring that the retirement income plan provides the flexibility and resources to pursue hobbies, travel, and other lifestyle goals

By taking a holistic approach and considering the interconnectedness of financial, physical, and psychological well-being, older adults can create a retirement plan that truly supports their overall quality of life.

Collaborating with a Trusted Financial Advisor

Navigating the complexities of retirement planning can be a daunting task, which is why it's crucial for older adults to work with a qualified, trusted financial advisor. A knowledgeable financial advisor can help:

- Develop a comprehensive retirement plan that addresses financial, health, and lifestyle goals
    - Provide guidance on investment strategies, tax planning, and risk management
    - Recommend appropriate insurance products, such as life, health, and

long-term care coverage
  - Coordinate with other healthcare providers and professionals to ensure a seamless, integrated approach to retirement planning

By collaborating with a financial advisor who takes a holistic, client-centered approach, older adults can feel empowered to make informed decisions and create a retirement plan that aligns with their unique needs and priorities.

Embracing Flexibility and Adaptability

Retirement planning is not a one-time event, but rather an ongoing process that requires flexibility and adaptability. As older adults navigate the various stages of retirement, their financial, physical, and emotional needs may evolve, necessitating periodic reviews and adjustments to their retirement plan.

By maintaining an open and adaptable mindset, older adults can:

- Regularly reassess their retirement goals and priorities as circumstances change
  - Make necessary modifications to their investment strategies, withdrawal plans, and insurance coverage
  - Explore new opportunities and adjust their lifestyle and spending as needed to maintain financial security and overall well-being

This commitment to flexibility and continuous improvement can help ensure that an older adult's retirement plan remains aligned with their evolving needs and supports their healthy aging journey.

Embracing the Financial Empowerment of Healthy Aging

As we have explored in this chapter, financial planning and retirement are essential components of the healthy aging journey. By taking a proactive, comprehensive approach to managing our financial resources, we can not only ensure a secure and independent retirement, but also support our physical, emotional, and social well-being throughout the golden years.

Remember, the path to financial security is not a one-size-fits-all endeavor. Each individual's needs, goals, and circumstances may vary, requiring a tailored and adaptable approach. By working closely with qualified financial advisors, healthcare providers, and trusted support networks, older adults can develop a personalized retirement plan that addresses their unique priorities and sets them up for long-term success.

Embracing financial empowerment is not just about the numbers and the bottom line – it's about creating the conditions for a fulfilling, independent, and resilient future. By taking control of our financial well-being, we can free ourselves to focus on the things that truly matter: maintaining our health, nurturing our relationships, and pursuing the activities and experiences that bring us joy and purpose.

As you embark on this financial planning journey, be patient, persistent, and open to learning. Celebrate your successes, learn from any setbacks, and remain flexible in your approach, as your needs and priorities may evolve over time. Remember that you are not alone in this process – reach out to your support networks, financial advisors, and the larger community of older adults who are committed to achieving financial security and overall well-being.

Ultimately, the financial empowerment of healthy aging is about more than just money – it's about creating the foundation for a life well-lived. By taking a proactive, holistic approach to retirement planning, we can unlock a world of possibilities and set an inspiring example for future generations. So, let's dive in, explore the financial strategies and resources that resonate most with you, and embrace the transformative power of financial security and healthy aging.

CHAPTER 12

Chapter 12: Caregiving and Support Systems

As we navigate the journey of healthy aging, it's important to recognize that we are not alone. At various stages of our lives, we may find ourselves in the role of caregiver, caring for a spouse, family member, or friend. Conversely, we may also require the support and assistance of caregivers as we face our own health challenges or changing needs.

In this chapter, we will explore the critical role of caregiving and support systems in the context of healthy aging. We will delve into the unique emotional, physical, and practical considerations for both caregivers and care recipients, and discuss strategies for building a strong, sustainable support network that empowers older adults to maintain their independence, well-being, and quality of life.

The Importance of Caregiving and Support Systems

Caregiving, whether provided by family members, friends, or professional services, plays a vital role in supporting the health, independence, and overall quality of life of older adults. By addressing the various needs of care recipients, caregivers can help to:

Maintain Independence and Daily Function

As we age, we may face increasing difficulties with activities of daily living, such as bathing, dressing, or managing medications. Caregiving support can help older adults continue living independently in their homes and communities, reducing the need for institutionalized care.

Manage Chronic Health Conditions

Many older adults live with one or more chronic health conditions, such as dementia, Parkinson's disease, or heart disease. Caregivers can assist with medication management, coordinating healthcare services, and implementing strategies to address the unique needs and symptoms associated with these conditions.

Enhance Emotional and Social Well-being

Caregiving can also play a crucial role in supporting the emotional and social well-being of older adults. Caregivers can provide companionship, engage in meaningful activities, and help maintain social connections, all of which can combat feelings of loneliness and isolation.

Prevent or Delay Institutional Care

By providing the necessary support and assistance, caregiving can help older adults avoid or delay the need for more intensive institutional care, such as nursing homes or assisted living facilities. This can have a significant impact on their quality of life and financial security.

Support the Caregiver's Well-being

It's important to recognize that caregiving can be an extremely rewarding experience, but it can also be physically and emotionally demanding. Providing support and resources for caregivers is essential for maintaining their own health and well-being, which in turn benefits the care recipient.

Navigating the Challenges of Caregiving

Caregiving for an older adult, whether a family member or friend, can be a complex and multifaceted responsibility. It's important for caregivers to be aware of the potential challenges they may face and to have strategies in place to address them effectively.

Emotional and Psychological Strain

Caring for a loved one can be emotionally and psychologically taxing, with caregivers often experiencing a range of complex emotions, such as:

- Stress, anxiety, and burnout
    - Feelings of guilt, resentment, or sadness
    - Grief over the changes in their loved one's health or abilities

Caregivers must prioritize their own emotional well-being and seek support to manage these challenges and prevent caregiver burnout.

Physical Demands and Health Risks

Caregiving can also take a physical toll, with caregivers often experiencing:

- Musculoskeletal injuries from assisting with physical tasks, such as lifting or transferring the care recipient
    - Disruptions to their own sleep, nutrition, and exercise routines
    - An increased risk of chronic health conditions, such as heart disease or diabetes

It's essential for caregivers to maintain their own physical health and well-being, which may require adaptations to their caregiving tasks or the use of assistive devices.

Financial and Practical Considerations

Caring for an older adult can also present significant financial and practical challenges, including:

- The cost of healthcare, medical equipment, or in-home care services
  - Reduced income due to the need to take time off work or reduce work hours
  - Navigating the complex landscape of insurance, government benefits, and community resources

Caregivers must be proactive in managing these practical and financial aspects of caregiving to ensure the well-being of both the care recipient and themselves.

Balancing Caregiving with Other Responsibilities

Many caregivers, particularly those in the "sandwich generation" who are caring for both older adults and children, must also juggle a range of other responsibilities, such as:

- Maintaining employment and managing work-life balance
  - Caring for their own children or grandchildren
  - Attending to their own personal and social needs

Striking a balance between caregiving and these other responsibilities can be extremely challenging, requiring careful planning, communication, and the utilization of available support systems.

Building a Comprehensive Support Network

To address the multifaceted challenges of caregiving and ensure the well-being of both the care recipient and the caregiver, it's essential to build a comprehensive support network. This network should include a combination of family members, friends, professional caregivers, and community resources.

Involving Family and Friends

The involvement of family members and close friends can be invaluable in providing both practical and emotional support for caregivers. Some ways to engage family and friends include:

- Establishing a care plan and dividing responsibilities among willing and able family members
    - Encouraging regular check-ins, visits, and assistance with tasks or errands
    - Organizing a support group or regular check-in meetings to share experiences and coping strategies

By cultivating this network of family and friends, caregivers can reduce the burden of their responsibilities and ensure that the care recipient receives the attention and support they need.

Utilizing Professional Caregiving Services

In addition to family and friends, professional caregiving services can also be an essential component of a comprehensive support network. These services may include:

- In-home care providers, such as home health aides or personal care assistants
    - Skilled nursing or rehabilitation services, for more complex medical needs
    - Adult day programs or respite care services, to provide temporary relief for the primary caregiver

By incorporating professional caregiving services into the support network, caregivers can ensure that the care recipient's needs are met, while also taking much-needed breaks to attend to their own well-being.

Accessing Community Resources and Support Groups

Beyond family, friends, and professional caregivers, older adults and their caregivers can also benefit from connecting with various community resources and support groups, such as:

- Local caregiver support groups, either in-person or virtual, to share experiences and coping strategies
  - Educational workshops or training programs on caregiving skills, self-care, and navigating the healthcare system
  - Volunteer programs or social activities that provide opportunities for the care recipient to engage with the community
  - Government or non-profit organizations that offer assistance, resources, or financial aid for caregivers and care recipients

By tapping into these community-based resources, caregivers can access valuable information, emotional support, and practical assistance to help them navigate the caregiving journey.

Developing a Care Plan and Maintaining Open Communication

Regardless of the specific support network, it's essential for caregivers and care recipients to work together to develop a comprehensive care plan that addresses the unique needs, preferences, and goals of the care recipient. This plan should include:

- A clear understanding of the care recipient's health status, care needs, and personal preferences
  - A schedule of caregiving responsibilities and the involvement of various support providers

- Strategies for managing medications, medical appointments, and health-care coordination
   - Contingency plans for emergencies or unexpected changes in the care recipient's condition

Maintaining open and transparent communication among all members of the support network is crucial for ensuring the effectiveness of the care plan and addressing any evolving needs or concerns.

Caring for the Caregiver: Strategies for Self-Care and Respite

While building a comprehensive support network is essential for the well-being of the care recipient, it's equally important to prioritize the self-care and respite needs of the caregiver. Caregivers who neglect their own physical, emotional, and social well-being are at a higher risk of burnout, which can ultimately compromise the quality of care they provide.

Prioritizing Physical and Emotional Well-being

Caregivers must be vigilant in maintaining their own physical and emotional health, which may include:

- Engaging in regular exercise, healthy eating, and adequate sleep
   - Practicing stress management techniques, such as meditation or mindfulness
   - Seeking professional counseling or support groups to manage the emotional challenges of caregiving

By prioritizing their own well-being, caregivers can better manage the demands of their role and prevent the negative impacts of caregiver burnout.

Scheduling Respite and Breaks

Caregivers should also make a concerted effort to schedule regular breaks and respite care, which can provide them with the opportunity to recharge, pursue their own interests, and avoid social isolation. Respite care options may include:

- In-home care services, such as home health aides or personal care assistants
    - Adult day programs or community-based respite services
    - Short-term stays in assisted living or nursing facilities

By incorporating regular respite into their routines, caregivers can maintain their energy, reduce the risk of burnout, and ensure they are able to provide high-quality care for their loved ones.

Seeking Support from Family, Friends, and Community

In addition to self-care and respite, caregivers can also benefit from the emotional and practical support of their family, friends, and broader community. This may involve:

- Asking family members or friends to assist with specific caregiving tasks or errands
    - Joining caregiver support groups, either in-person or online, to share experiences and coping strategies
    - Engaging with community organizations or faith-based groups that offer resources and services for caregivers

By tapping into these sources of support, caregivers can reduce their sense of isolation, gain new insights and strategies, and maintain their own well-being throughout the caregiving journey.

Preparing for the Transition of Care

As older adults and their caregivers navigate the various stages of the caregiving journey, there may come a time when the care recipient's needs exceed the capabilities of the existing support network. This transition of care, such as the move to an assisted living facility or nursing home, can be a challenging and emotionally charged experience for both the care recipient and the caregiver.

Engaging in Advance Care Planning

To prepare for potential changes in the care recipient's needs, it's essential to engage in advance care planning. This process involves:

- Discussing the care recipient's preferences, values, and goals for their care
  - Documenting legal documents, such as a living will or power of attorney, to ensure their wishes are honored
  - Identifying the triggers or thresholds that may necessitate a transition of care

By proactively addressing these considerations, caregivers and care recipients can feel more informed and empowered to make decisions that align with the care recipient's values and priorities.

Navigating the Transition of Care

When the time comes to transition the care recipient to a new living situation or level of care, caregivers should:

- Involve the care recipient in the decision-making process, to the extent possible, and validate their feelings about the transition
  - Research and evaluate potential care providers, such as assisted living facilities or nursing homes, to find the best fit
  - Coordinate the logistics of the move, including packing, transportation, and the transfer of medical records
  - Maintain regular communication and involvement with the new care

providers to ensure a smooth transition and continuity of care

Throughout this process, caregivers should also prioritize their own self-care and emotional well-being, as the transition can be particularly challenging and draining.

Providing Ongoing Support and Advocacy

Even after a transition of care, the caregiver's role often continues, albeit in a different capacity. Caregivers can continue to provide support by:

- Maintaining regular visits and communication with the care recipient
  - Advocating for the care recipient's needs and preferences with the new care providers
  - Assisting with medical appointments, care coordination, and financial management
  - Providing emotional support and helping the care recipient adapt to their new living situation

By remaining engaged and advocating for the care recipient's well-being, caregivers can help ensure a smooth and successful transition, while also maintaining their own sense of purpose and involvement in the caregiving journey.

Embracing the Transformative Power of Caregiving and Support Systems

As we have explored in this chapter, the role of caregiving and support systems is a critical component of healthy aging. By building a comprehensive network of support, caregivers and care recipients can navigate the challenges of aging with resilience, independence, and a renewed sense of purpose.

Remember, the caregiving journey is not a solitary one – it requires the collaboration, understanding, and support of a diverse array of individuals and community resources. By reaching out to family, friends, professionals, and the broader community, both caregivers and care recipients can access the information, assistance, and emotional support they need to thrive.

For caregivers, it's essential to recognize the importance of self-care and respite. By prioritizing their own physical, emotional, and social well-being, they can better manage the demands of their role and prevent burnout, ultimately enhancing the quality of care they provide.

For care recipients, the support network can be a lifeline, empowering them to maintain their independence, address their healthcare needs, and continue participating in the activities and relationships that bring them joy and fulfillment.

Ultimately, the transformative power of caregiving and support systems lies in the creation of a collaborative, adaptive, and resilient approach to healthy aging. By embracing this comprehensive, community-based model of care, we can redefine the narrative of aging, inspire and empower those around us, and demonstrate the incredible value that caregiving and support can bring to the lives of older adults.

So, let's embark on this journey together, drawing upon the strategies, resources, and insights outlined in this chapter. Whether you find yourself in the role of caregiver or care recipient, remember that you are not alone. Reach out, connect with others, and unlock the boundless potential of a strong, supportive network that empowers you to live your best life in the golden years and beyond.

CHAPTER 13

hapter 13: Lifelong Learning and Personal Growth

C As we navigate the journey of healthy aging, it's essential to recognize that our growth and development do not stop once we reach a certain age. The golden years can be a time of profound personal transformation, intellectual stimulation, and continued learning - all of which can have a profound impact on our overall well-being, independence, and quality of life.

In this chapter, we will explore the importance of embracing a lifelong learning mindset and incorporating opportunities for personal growth into our daily lives. We will delve into the cognitive, emotional, and social benefits of continuous learning, and discuss practical strategies for cultivating a growth-oriented mindset and engaging in enriching activities that support our unique interests and goals.

By the end of this chapter, you will be equipped with the knowledge and inspiration to embark on a transformative journey of lifelong learning and personal development, empowering you to thrive in the golden years and beyond.

The Cognitive Benefits of Lifelong Learning

Maintaining an active, engaged mind is crucial for preserving cognitive function and delaying age-related cognitive decline. Engaging in lifelong learning activities can provide a wealth of benefits for older adults, including:

Enhancing Neuroplasticity and Cognitive Flexibility

The human brain is a remarkably adaptable organ, with the capacity to change, grow, and reorganize itself throughout our lives. This ability, known as neuroplasticity, is the foundation for learning and the acquisition of new skills and knowledge.

By consistently challenging ourselves with novel intellectual activities, such as learning a new language, playing strategic games, or exploring creative pursuits, we can stimulate the formation of new neural connections and strengthen existing ones. This, in turn, can enhance our cognitive flexibility, problem-solving abilities, and overall mental agility, helping us adapt more effectively to the changes and challenges that often come with aging.

Improving Memory and Information Processing

Engaging in lifelong learning can also have a direct impact on our memory and information processing abilities. As we age, we may experience gradual declines in certain cognitive functions, such as short-term memory or the speed at which we process new information.

However, research has shown that older adults who regularly participate in mentally stimulating activities, such as taking classes, reading, or engaging in discussion groups, can experience improvements in their memory performance and information processing speed. This can translate to better everyday functioning, improved decision-making, and a greater sense of confidence and independence.

Reducing the Risk of Cognitive Decline and Dementia

In addition to the immediate cognitive benefits, lifelong learning has also been associated with a reduced risk of age-related cognitive decline and the development of dementia, including Alzheimer's disease. By continuously challenging the brain and maintaining an active, engaged lifestyle, older adults can potentially delay the onset of these debilitating conditions and preserve their cognitive abilities for longer.

This protective effect is thought to be the result of the brain's ability to build cognitive reserve, a concept that suggests the more we challenge our minds, the more adaptable and resilient our brains become in the face of age-related changes or neurological damage.

The Emotional and Social Benefits of Lifelong Learning

In addition to the cognitive advantages, embracing a lifelong learning mindset can also have a profound impact on our emotional well-being and social connections, both of which are essential for healthy aging.

Enhancing Emotional Well-being and Resilience

Engaging in lifelong learning activities can have a positive influence on our emotional state and overall psychological resilience. The sense of accomplishment, mastery, and personal growth that comes from acquiring new skills or knowledge can boost our self-esteem, confidence, and feelings of purpose.

Moreover, the social interactions and intellectual stimulation inherent in many learning activities can help combat feelings of loneliness, depression, and anxiety, which are common challenges for older adults. By nurturing our emotional well-being through lifelong learning, we can better navigate the physical, social, and psychological changes that often occur in the golden years.

Fostering Social Connections and Engagement

Lifelong learning can also serve as a powerful tool for building and maintaining social connections, a crucial aspect of healthy aging. Participating in educational classes, discussion groups, or other learning-based activities provides older adults with opportunities to meet new people, exchange ideas, and engage in meaningful discussions.

These social interactions not only combat feelings of isolation but can also lead to the formation of new friendships and the strengthening of existing relationships. By staying socially engaged and intellectually stimulated, older adults can maintain a sense of belonging, purpose, and community, all of which contribute to their overall well-being and quality of life.

Encouraging Continued Personal Growth and Fulfillment

Embracing a lifelong learning mindset can also foster a sense of ongoing personal growth and fulfillment. As we age, we may find ourselves with more time and resources to explore new interests, pursue passions, or develop skills that we were unable to focus on earlier in life.

By continuously challenging ourselves and stepping outside of our comfort zones, we can experience a renewed sense of excitement, curiosity, and self-discovery. This can lead to a greater sense of purpose, a more positive outlook on aging, and a heightened appreciation for the richness and diversity of our life experiences.

Strategies for Embracing Lifelong Learning

Incorporating lifelong learning into our daily lives can take many forms, from formal educational programs to informal self-directed activities. The key is to find approaches that align with our personal interests, learning styles, and lifestyle preferences.

Formal Educational Programs and Courses

Older adults have access to a wide range of formal educational opportunities, both in-person and online, that can provide structured learning experiences and the chance to interact with peers and instructors. Some options to consider include:

- Continuing education classes or adult learning programs through local colleges, universities, or community colleges
  - Specialized certification or skills-based training programs, such as those offered through professional associations or industry organizations
  - Lifelong learning institutes or programs designed specifically for older adults, which often offer a diverse curriculum and social activities

By engaging in these formal educational programs, older adults can not only acquire new knowledge and skills but also benefit from the social connections and sense of community that they foster.

Informal Self-directed Learning

In addition to structured educational programs, older adults can also pursue self-directed learning opportunities that align with their personal interests and goals. These informal learning activities may include:

- Reading books, magazines, or online articles on topics of interest
  - Watching educational documentaries, online lectures, or video tutorials
  - Participating in discussion groups, book clubs, or online forums
  - Exploring creative hobbies, such as art, music, or writing
  - Engaging in hands-on activities, such as gardening, woodworking, or cooking

The beauty of self-directed learning is that it allows older adults to tailor their educational experiences to their unique preferences and learning styles, fostering a sense of autonomy, curiosity, and personal fulfillment.

Intergenerational Learning Opportunities

As part of their lifelong learning journey, older adults can also benefit from engaging in intergenerational learning experiences. These opportunities allow them to share their knowledge, wisdom, and life experiences with younger generations, while also learning from the unique perspectives and skills of their younger counterparts.

Some examples of intergenerational learning activities include:

- Volunteering as a tutor or mentor in local schools or community programs
    - Participating in joint projects or workshops with younger participants
    - Engaging in storytelling or oral history initiatives to preserve cultural knowledge
    - Collaborating on creative or entrepreneurial ventures that leverage the strengths of different age groups

By bridging the generational gap through learning and shared experiences, older adults can cultivate a sense of purpose, strengthen their social connections, and contribute to the personal growth and development of others.

Utilizing Technology and Online Resources

In the digital age, older adults have access to a vast array of online resources and technologies that can facilitate their lifelong learning journey. From educational platforms and virtual classes to social media groups and online communities, the possibilities for engaging in self-directed and collaborative learning are endless.

Some examples of how older adults can leverage technology for lifelong learning include:

- Enrolling in online courses or MOOCs (Massive Open Online Courses) offered by universities or educational providers
  - Participating in virtual discussion groups, webinars, or video-based learning experiences
  - Connecting with like-minded individuals through social media groups or online forums
  - Utilizing productivity apps, language-learning software, or brain-training exercises to continuously challenge the mind

By embracing technology and online resources, older adults can overcome geographic barriers, access a wealth of educational content, and engage in flexible, self-paced learning that fits seamlessly into their daily routines.

Cultivating a Growth Mindset for Healthy Aging

At the core of lifelong learning and personal growth is the adoption of a growth mindset - a belief that our abilities and intelligence are not fixed, but can be developed and improved through dedication, effort, and a willingness to learn from challenges.

Embracing a growth mindset is particularly important in the context of healthy aging, as it can help older adults approach the changes and transitions of later life with a sense of resilience, adaptability, and continuous improvement.

Fostering a Positive Attitude Towards Aging

One of the key components of a growth mindset for healthy aging is the cultivation of a positive attitude towards the aging process. Rather than viewing age as a limitation or a barrier to growth, older adults with a growth mindset see the golden years as an opportunity to explore new possibilities, challenge themselves, and continue on a journey of self-discovery.

This positive mindset can help older adults approach age-related changes, such as physical or cognitive changes, with a sense of curiosity and a willingness to adapt, rather than resignation or fear. By embracing the idea that they can continue to learn, grow, and improve, even in the face of adversity, older adults can maintain a sense of control, purpose, and overall well-being.

Cultivating a Lifelong Learning Mindset

In addition to a positive attitude towards aging, a growth mindset for healthy aging also involves the cultivation of a lifelong learning mindset. This mindset is characterized by a deep curiosity, a willingness to take risks, and a commitment to continuous improvement and personal development.

Older adults with a lifelong learning mindset are not content to simply maintain the status quo or coast through their golden years. Instead, they actively seek out new challenges, embrace feedback and constructive criticism, and view setbacks as opportunities for growth and learning.

By nurturing this lifelong learning mindset, older adults can stay engaged, motivated, and intellectually stimulated, ultimately enhancing their cognitive function, emotional well-being, and overall quality of life.

Embracing Adaptability and Resilience

Finally, a growth mindset for healthy aging also encompasses the ability to adapt to change and maintain resilience in the face of adversity. As we age, we inevitably encounter various transitions and challenges, such as changes in health, relationships, or living situations.

Older adults with a growth mindset approach these changes not with fear or resistance, but with a willingness to learn, adjust, and find new ways to thrive. They understand that growth and personal development are not linear processes, but rather involve ups and downs, successes and failures.

By cultivating adaptability and resilience, older adults can navigate the complexities of aging with a sense of confidence, empowerment, and a deep appreciation for the richness and diversity of their life experiences.

Embracing the Transformative Power of Lifelong Learning and Personal Growth

As we have explored in this chapter, embracing lifelong learning and personal growth is a powerful and transformative approach to healthy aging. By continuously challenging our minds, nurturing our emotional well-being, and fostering a growth mindset, we can unlock a world of benefits that can enhance our physical, cognitive, and social well-being throughout the golden years and beyond.

Remember, the journey of lifelong learning and personal growth is not a solitary one – it involves the exploration of new ideas, the exchange of perspectives, and the cultivation of meaningful connections with others. By engaging with educational programs, online resources, and intergenerational learning opportunities, older adults can build a vibrant network of support, inspiration, and shared experiences.

Moreover, embracing lifelong learning and personal growth is not just about the individual – it's about creating a ripple effect that can inspire and empower others. By sharing our knowledge, skills, and life experiences with younger generations, older adults can leave a lasting legacy and contribute to the personal growth and development of their communities.

As you embark on this transformative journey, be patient, persistent, and open to new experiences. Celebrate your successes, learn from your setbacks, and remain flexible in your approach, as your interests and goals may evolve over time. Remember that you are not alone in this process – reach out to your support networks, educational institutions, and the larger community of lifelong learners who are committed to personal growth and healthy aging.

Ultimately, the power of lifelong learning and personal growth lies in its ability to unlock our boundless potential, enhance our overall well-being, and create a more vibrant, engaged, and interconnected society. By embracing this mindset and incorporating it into our daily lives, we can redefine the aging experience and demonstrate the incredible transformative power of continuous learning and self-discovery.

So, let's dive in, explore the educational and personal growth opportunities that resonate most with you, and embark on a journey of intellectual stimulation, emotional fulfillment, and lasting legacy. The future is bright, and it starts with a curious, growth-oriented mindset that celebrates the richness and diversity of our life experiences.

CONCLUSION

As we reach the final chapter of our journey through the Healthy Aging Handbook, it's important to reflect on the incredible transformation and personal growth we have experienced. The path of healthy aging is not merely about maintaining physical health or delaying the onset of age-related diseases – it's about embracing a holistic approach that nurtures our physical, cognitive, emotional, and social well-being, empowering us to live our golden years with purpose, resilience, and a deep appreciation for the richness of our lives.

In this culminating chapter, we will explore the art of celebrating healthy aging and the powerful legacy we can leave behind. We will delve into the positive aspects of growing older, the importance of finding meaning and purpose, and the profound impact we can have on our families, communities, and future generations.

By embracing this celebratory and legacy-driven mindset, we can not only enhance our own quality of life but also inspire and empower others to embark on their own transformative journeys of healthy aging.

Embracing the Positive Aspects of Aging

While the common narrative surrounding aging often focuses on the challenges and losses associated with growing older, it's essential to recognize and celebrate the myriad of positive aspects that can come with this stage of life. By shifting our perspective and embracing the unique gifts and opportunities of the golden years, we can cultivate a profound sense of gratitude, purpose, and personal fulfillment.

Greater Emotional Maturity and Wisdom

As we age, we often develop a deeper emotional intelligence and wisdom that can serve as a guiding light for ourselves and those around us. Through the accumulation of life experiences, both joyful and challenging, we gain a nuanced understanding of human nature, the complexities of relationships, and the ebb and flow of emotions.

This emotional maturity can translate into greater empathy, patience, and the ability to navigate personal and interpersonal challenges with a heightened sense of perspective and grace. By sharing this wisdom with others, we can serve as mentors, sounding boards, and sources of comfort and support, enriching the lives of those we encounter.

Increased Confidence and Self-Acceptance

Another positive aspect of aging is the growing sense of confidence and self-acceptance that often accompanies the later stages of life. As we shed the insecurities and self-consciousness that may have defined our younger years, we can embrace our authentic selves with greater ease and authenticity.

This increased self-assurance can empower us to take risks, pursue new passions, and unapologetically express our unique perspectives and values. By embodying this self-acceptance, we can inspire others to cultivate their own confidence and live more fulfilling, self-directed lives.

Freedom and Flexibility

The transition into retirement and the golden years can also bring a newfound sense of freedom and flexibility that may have been elusive during our working years. With fewer constraints on our time and a reduced need to adhere to rigid schedules or external obligations, we can explore new hobbies, travel, and engage in activities that truly resonate with our interests and values.

This freedom can foster a greater sense of personal autonomy, allowing us to curate our daily lives in a way that nourishes our well-being and brings us joy. By embracing this flexibility, we can design our golden years in a way that aligns with our evolving needs and aspirations, creating a more fulfilling and rewarding experience.

Deepening of Relationships and Connections

As we grow older, we often have the opportunity to deepen our existing relationships and forge new, meaningful connections with others. With more time and emotional resources to devote to our loved ones, we can cultivate richer, more profound bonds that transcend the superficial interactions of our younger years.

This deepening of relationships can provide a profound sense of belonging, support, and shared experiences, all of which contribute to our overall emotional well-being and quality of life. By nurturing these connections, we can create a strong foundation of love and support that sustains us throughout the golden years and beyond.

Finding Meaning and Purpose in the Golden Years

As we embrace the positive aspects of aging, it's equally important to cultivate a sense of meaning and purpose in our lives. By identifying the activities, relationships, and contributions that bring us a profound sense of fulfillment, we can design a retirement and later-life experience that is deeply satisfying and aligned with our core values.

Pursuing Passions and Lifelong Interests

One of the joys of the golden years is the opportunity to dedicate more time and energy to the hobbies, creative pursuits, and lifelong interests that may have been sidelined during our working lives. Whether it's delving into a new artistic medium, exploring the great outdoors, or mastering a long-desired skill, engaging in these passions can provide a profound sense of purpose and personal growth.

By immersing ourselves in activities that ignite our curiosity and creative spark, we can experience a renewed sense of vitality, self-expression, and overall well-being. These pursuits not only enrich our own lives but can also inspire and engage others, creating a ripple effect of positivity and inspiration.

Volunteering and Community Involvement

Another powerful way to find meaning and purpose in the golden years is through volunteer work and community involvement. By dedicating our time and talents to causes, organizations, or initiatives that align with our values, we can make a tangible difference in the lives of others while simultaneously nurturing our own sense of purpose and fulfillment.

Volunteering opportunities can range from providing educational support to children, to assisting at local food banks, to advocating for environmental conservation. Regardless of the specific focus, these community-based engagements allow us to leverage our unique skills and life experiences to benefit others, create lasting change, and leave a positive legacy.

Mentoring and Intergenerational Connections

In addition to volunteering, the golden years also present an opportunity to mentor and share our wisdom with younger generations. By engaging in intergenerational learning and teaching experiences, we can pass on our hard-earned knowledge, insights, and life lessons to those who can benefit from our perspective and guidance.

Whether it's tutoring students, coaching younger professionals, or imparting our accumulated wisdom to family members, the act of mentoring can provide a profound sense of purpose and the gratification of positively impacting the lives of others. Furthermore, these intergenerational connections can foster a greater sense of community, mutual understanding, and continued personal growth for all involved.

Leaving a Lasting Legacy

Ultimately, the process of finding meaning and purpose in the golden years is not just about fulfilling our own desires and aspirations – it's about creating a lasting legacy that will endure long after we are gone. By dedicating our time, talents, and resources to causes and initiatives that are greater than ourselves, we can leave an indelible mark on the world and inspire future generations to continue on the path of healthy aging and positive transformation.

This legacy can take many forms, from establishing charitable foundations or scholarships, to authoring books or creating works of art, to advocating for social or environmental change. Regardless of the specific manifestation, the act of legacy-building allows us to transcend the limitations of our own lifespan and contribute to the ongoing betterment of our communities and the world at large.

Embracing the Celebratory Spirit of Healthy Aging

As we have explored the positive aspects of aging and the pursuit of meaning and purpose, it's essential to also recognize the importance of celebration – the act of embracing and honoring the unique gifts and achievements of the golden years. By cultivating a celebratory mindset, we can not only enhance our own quality of life but also inspire and empower others to embark on their own transformative journeys of healthy aging.

Celebrating Milestones and Accomplishments

One of the fundamental ways to celebrate healthy aging is to acknowledge and commemorate the various milestones and accomplishments that we reach along the way. Whether it's the attainment of a new skill, the completion of a personal goal, or the achievement of a significant birthday or anniversary, these moments deserve to be recognized and celebrated with a sense of pride, joy, and gratitude.

By taking the time to honor these milestones, we not only reinforce our sense of personal growth and achievement but also create opportunities to gather with loved ones, share our experiences, and deepen our connections with one another. This celebratory spirit can serve as a powerful motivator, encouraging us to continue pursuing our passions and personal development throughout the golden years.

Fostering a Culture of Positivity and Inspiration

Beyond individual celebrations, it's also essential to cultivate a broader culture of positivity and inspiration around the concept of healthy aging. By sharing our stories, successes, and lessons learned with our families, communities, and the world at large, we can challenge the negative stereotypes and misconceptions that often surround the aging process.

This can involve actively participating in public conversations, writing for local publications, or engaging in social media initiatives that showcase the vibrant, fulfilling, and purposeful nature of the golden years. By amplifying these positive narratives, we can inspire others to reframe their own perceptions of aging and embrace the incredible transformative potential of healthy aging.

Celebrating the Richness of Life Experiences

Ultimately, the most profound way to celebrate healthy aging is to embrace and honor the rich tapestry of life experiences that have brought us to this point. From the triumphs and challenges of our younger years to the wisdom and self-actualization of the golden age, each phase of our lives has contributed to the unique individuals we have become.

By reflecting on and celebrating this lifetime of growth, resilience, and personal evolution, we can cultivate a deep sense of gratitude, pride, and appreciation for the extraordinary journey of our lives. This celebratory mindset not only enhances our own well-being but also serves as a powerful inspiration for those around us, demonstrating the incredible transformative potential of healthy aging.

Leaving a Lasting Legacy

As we near the end of our journey through the Healthy Aging Handbook, it's important to recognize that the legacy we leave behind is not just about the material possessions or financial assets we accumulated over the course of our lives. Rather, our true legacy lies in the positive impact we have had on the lives of others, the wisdom and values we have imparted, and the inspiring example we have set for future generations.

Passing on Values and Wisdom

One of the most enduring aspects of our legacy is the values, principles, and life lessons we have cultivated over the years. By actively sharing these insights with our loved ones, our communities, and the world at large, we can ensure that our most cherished beliefs and perspectives continue to shape the lives of others long after we are gone.

This can involve documenting our personal histories, recording our life stories, or engaging in dynamic conversations and teaching experiences that allow us to impart our hard-earned wisdom. Regardless of the specific approach, the act of passing on our values and insights can serve as a powerful testament to the richness and significance of our lives.

Inspiring and Empowering Others

Another crucial component of our legacy is the positive impact we have had on the lives of others. Whether it's through our roles as mentors, volunteers, or engaged community members, the ripple effects of our actions and the inspiration we have provided can continue to transform the world around us.

By embracing a spirit of service, generosity, and compassion, we can leave an indelible mark on the individuals and communities we have touched. This legacy of inspiration and empowerment can manifest in myriad ways, from the young professionals we have guided to the social causes we have championed to the families we have supported and nurtured.

Cultivating a Lasting Positive Change

Ultimately, the most enduring legacy we can leave behind is one of lasting positive change – the fundamental transformation of the world around us in ways that outlive our own existence. This can involve establishing charitable foundations, contributing to scientific or medical research, or advocating for important social or environmental causes.

By dedicating our time, resources, and passions to initiatives that address pressing global challenges, we can create a powerful legacy that continues to make a tangible difference long after we are gone. Whether it's advancing the frontiers of healthcare, championing the rights of marginalized communities, or safeguarding the health of our planet, these legacy-building efforts can serve as a testament to the profound impact we have had on the world.

Embracing the Boundless Potential of Healthy Aging

As we bring our journey through the Healthy Aging Handbook to a close, it's important to reflect on the incredible transformation and personal growth we have experienced. From enhancing our physical, cognitive, and emotional well-being to cultivating a sense of purpose, meaning, and legacy, we have unlocked the boundless potential of healthy aging.

Remember, the path of healthy aging is not a linear or solitary one – it's a dynamic, collaborative, and ever-evolving process that requires flexibility, adaptability, and a willingness to embrace new challenges and opportunities. By continuing to learn, grow, and celebrate the positive aspects of aging, we can not only enrich our own lives but also inspire and empower others to embark on their own transformative journeys.

Ultimately, the legacy we leave behind is not just about the material or financial assets we accumulate, but rather the positive impact we have had on the lives of others, the values and wisdom we have imparted, and the lasting change we have helped to create. By embracing a celebratory and legacy-driven mindset, we can transcend the limitations of our own lifespan and contribute to the ongoing betterment of our communities and the world at large.

So, as we close this chapter and look towards the boundless possibilities that await us, let us continue to embrace the power of healthy aging with a profound sense of gratitude, purpose, and inspiration. Let us celebrate our milestones, share our stories, and leave an indelible mark on the lives of those around us. Together, we can redefine the narrative of aging and demonstrate the transformative potential of living our golden years to the fullest.

The future is bright, and it starts with the decisions we make today. Let us continue on this journey, empowered, resilient, and filled with a deep appreciation for the richness and diversity of our life experiences. The world awaits, and our legacy is yet to be written.